Healthcare
Informatics

Healthcare Informatics

C. William Hanson III, MD

Professor of Anesthesiology and Critical Care,
Internal Medicine and Surgery
University of Pennsylvania, School of Medicine,
Philadelphia, Pennsylvania

Visiting Professor of Computer Science
Princeton University
Princeton, New Jersey

McGraw-Hill
Medical Publishing Division

New York • Chicago • San Francisco • Lisbon • London • Madrid
Mexico City • Milan • New Delhi • San Juan • Seoul
Singapore • Sydney • Toronto

The McGraw·Hill Companies

Healthcare Informatics

1 2 3 4 5 6 7 8 9 0   DOC/DOC   0 9 8 7 6 5

ISBN: 0-07-144066-6

This book was set in Sabon by International Typesetting and Composition, Inc.
The editors were James F. Shanahan, Robert Pancotti, and Peter J. Boyle.
The production supervisor was Catherine Saggese.
Project management was provided by International Typesetting and Composition, Inc.
The index was prepared by Stephen Ingle.
RR Donnelley was the printer and binder.

Library of Congress Cataloging-in-Publication Data

Hanson, C. William (Clarence William), 1955–
    Healthcare informatics / C. William Hanson III.
        p. cm.
    Includes bibliographical references and index.
    ISBN 0-07-144066-6 (alk. paper)
    1. Medical informatics. I. Title.

    R858.H38 2005
    610'.28—dc22   2005052243

*I dedicate this book to my family, Cal, Ad, Wat, and Beth,
from whom I borrowed too much time during its completion,
and to my dusty muse, whence the inspiration springs.*

CONTENTS

PREFACE

Computerization has come slowly to the medical industry, but it is now apparent that computers and medical informatics are essential to its survival. Given the largeness and complexity of modern health delivery, its regulatory and administrative burdens, and of course its financial pressures, it is inescapable that computers will be brought to bear throughout the system in every conceivable stage of patient care and management.

We are now 20 years into the era of the personal computer and somewhat less than that into the Internet era, which means that something like half of today's active health-care workers started their careers before computers had much to do with patient care. In addition, very few of the other, younger, half has had any formal training in computer science.

Physicians, nurses, and other healthcare professionals are commonly well versed in, and facile with, complex technology used in modern diagnostic and therapeutic medicine. Computers and informatics are oddly separated from this comfort zone. Given the industry's increasingly reliance on informatics, and the lack of familiarity among many health professionals with basic principles and fundamental applications, a primer of the essentials for non-IT specialists can serve a helpful purpose.

This book is designed to provide physicians, nurses, and ancillary medical workers with an introduction to computers and medical informatics as they relate to the clinical environment. The first half of the book is generally focused on topics having to do with computers and networking. The second half is more specifically focused on medically oriented topics and concludes with my vision of what the very near future holds in medical computing. Each chapter ends with a number of references for further investigation for readers so inclined.

C. William Hanson III, MD

ACKNOWLEDGMENTS

My thanks for belief in the concept for this book go to Jim Shanahan at McGraw-Hill. I would also like to acknowledge the friendship, education, and advice I've gotten from my colleagues in the computer science department at Princeton over the past several years and several others to whom I owe thanks:

Drs. Kai Li, Brian Kernighan, Tom Funkhouser, Perry Cook, Ed Felten, Larry Peterson, and David Dobkin.

Drs. Randy Miller, Ted Shortliffe, Mark Weiner, Don Rucker, and my old friend Jon Cohen for their help with the informatics course at Princeton that led to the development of the book.

Finally, I'd like to thank Drs. David Longnecker and Lee Fleisher for creating an environment at Penn that encourages projects of this sort.

1

Hardware: Anatomy and Physiology of a Personal Computer

Introduction

Several years ago our hospital installed new personal computers throughout patient care areas. The machines are used for order entry, patient tracking, lab and radiology information, literature searches, and Internet access. When they were initially installed, they were quiet. Today, however, many of them have developed a continuous, high-pitched whine. Many of the health care professionals who use these computers as a part of their daily activities don't have any idea what the noise might be. Some of them aren't aware of the fact that there are more moving parts in a computer than those associated with the floppy drive. Most of them are not aware that this noise might be a problem.

A computer is like a living organism in many ways. Its anatomy is relatively consistent across brands. Computers sicken, age, and eventually die. There are ways to diagnose illness in a computer that refer back to its parts and their function. Like a cardiac murmur, the whine in an aging computer can only come from a moving part. Since the whine is continuous, and continues when the floppy drive is not being accessed, it must originate from a part that is moving continuously. This can only be the cooling fan or the hard disk drive. If it is the hard disk drive, and it is a new or worsening sound, it may imply that the drive is at risk for a catastrophic failure and therefore loss of the data on the drive. While this may not be particularly interesting to the individual practitioner when the computer belongs to the hospital, it becomes much more compelling when you own the computer and its data.

This chapter describes the anatomy of a generic computer, what each part does and how it works. The information is sufficiently generic that it applies to virtually all PCs including those manufactured by Apple, IBM, Dell, and others.

Before starting any discussion about hardware, a brief discussion about how computers work is in order. Computers are made of electrical circuits that are designed to understand and do things based on binary numbers—numbers where each digit is either a 0 or a 1. In the computer a 0 is represented by one electrical voltage (3.3 V) and the 1 by another (5 V). Each binary digit is called a bit, and bits are grouped together in bytes (usually 8 bits long). Depending on the context, a byte can be used to represent a number, a character, a portion of an image or an instruction. Instructions are grouped together to make programs (like a word processing program) and programs operate on groups of data (like a text document). Computers are incredibly fast and many processes (e.g., video display management and word processing) are performed in parallel, but it all comes down to electrical bits moving around in an organized fashion through a machine (Fig. 1-1).

The Motherboard

Key Points

- The motherboard is the skeleton and nervous system of the computer.
- Basic input-output system (BIOS) contains start-up instructions.

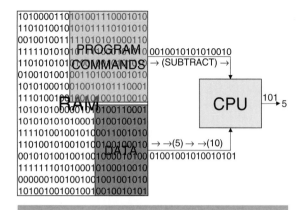

Figure 1-1
Programs and data are stored together in memory in the form of electronic bits, and the program commands direct the central processing unit in its management of the data.

- CMOS RAM contains information about the specific configuration of the computer and the computer's time.
- The chipset orchestrates the flow of instructions and data through the system.
- System memory consists of memory caches (short-term storage bins) and RAM.
- The system buses are the "highways" for the flow of data through the computer and vary in capacity.
- The central processing unit (CPU) is the engine of the computer and its speed depends on the capacity of its internal buses, its clock speed, and how efficient it is in executing instructions.

Motherboard Layout

The motherboard is analogous to the bony skeleton of a computer. It is a circuit board with a standardized layout (or anatomy) that determines where various components like the CPU are located. The specific layout for desktop PCs is described in an industry wide, open (i.e., nonproprietary) specification. The most common designs in use today are the AT (as in the old IBM PC/AT) and the newer ATX formats (there is an even newer BTX format that is just coming into the market).

The AT format predominated through the middle 1990s and the ATX format, which was introduced in the late 1990s, is used in all new computers. The newer (ATX) format was modified in a number of ways such as the relocation of insertion points for devices. It was also rotated relative to the AT layout to accommodate smaller expansion boards (like the video and network boards that plug into the motherboard), facilitate cooling of the CPU, and address new memory standards (Fig. 1-2).

The motherboard has evolved over time. Early motherboards were directly analogous to the biological spine and central nervous system in that they were primarily designed for signal communication across "buses," with rigid attachment points for

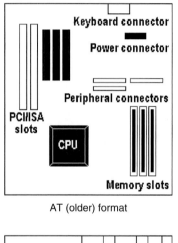

AT (older) format

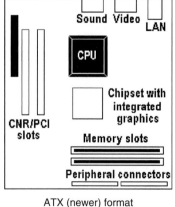

ATX (newer) format

Figure 1-2
AT vs. ATX motherboard format.

"appendicular" devices including the power supply and the CPU. The components that controlled video display and the disk drives were removably attached to the motherboard using plug-in slots. Newer motherboards using the ATX footprint are often equipped with *built-in* components—video, sound, network communications, and hard and floppy drive control are often built directly into the motherboard. The downside to this approach relates to devices that evolve rapidly (e.g., graphics). Since they are hard-wired to the motherboard, they cannot be upgraded independently as new capabilities become available. Conversely, some users may not need some of the (costly) functions (e.g., network communications) built into a given motherboard.

BIOS

All motherboards have a small, built-in block of read-only (nonwritable) memory, the BIOS, or basic input-output system that contains the instructions for starting-up, self-checking, and the initial communication with devices such as the CD and hard disk drives (Fig. 1-3). Once this initial phase is complete, the BIOS program looks for an *operating system* (such as the Mac OS, one of the Windows families or Linux). It checks the floppy drive, hard disk drive, and CD-ROM in a predetermined sequence. This process is known as *booting up* and is derived from the expression "to pull oneself up by one's bootstraps," referring to the fact that a small amount of computer code (the bootstrap) loads successively larger chunks of code, which then run the computer. This process will be discussed more extensively in Chap. 2.

The CMOS RAM

Another area of the motherboard has a small block of writable memory powered by a battery. This is called the CMOS (complementary metal oxide silicon) RAM (random access memory). This area stores information about the computer's configuration and the reference time (usually today's time and date), in the real time clock (RTC). The computer checks this time when it powers up and then keeps its own time using the CPU while the computer is running. Because the RTC is battery powered, it maintains a current version of the time even when the computer is off.

The Chipset

The chipset is a group of circuits that act as traffic cops, orchestrating the flow of information among the various components of the computer including the CPU, various memory locations, I/O (input-output) devices (i.e., mouse, keyboard), and peripherals (i.e., network cards, video, and so on).

On-board Memory (Caches and RAM)

PC memory comes in a variety of flavors representing tradeoffs among speed, size, and cost. One would ideally like to have an enormous amount of extremely fast memory directly available to the processor. Improvements in processor speed have significantly outstripped improvements in memory speed in the past decade, and without well-designed memory architectures, the processor would sit idle waiting for data from memory for much of the time. The solution that has been implemented on today's PCs is to use a series of data *caches* as holding pens for data that are likely to be needed in the near future by the processor.

A typical modern architecture includes a primary cache, or level 1 (L1) cache, on the processor itself. A secondary, or level 2 (L2), cache is located on the motherboard adjacent to the CPU (on the newest processors the L2 cache may be on the processor as well). Cache memory is implemented in *static random access memory* (SRAM), which is faster and more expensive than *dynamic random access memory* (DRAM). DRAM is used for main memory, or what's typically referred to as RAM.

Caching improves performance by keeping recently accessed data or instructions (or those that are likely to be requested) in faster memory nearer the processor. A mental model of how this works is as follows. A central section of *program code instructions* (from a word processor program for example) and a block of *data* (pages from a

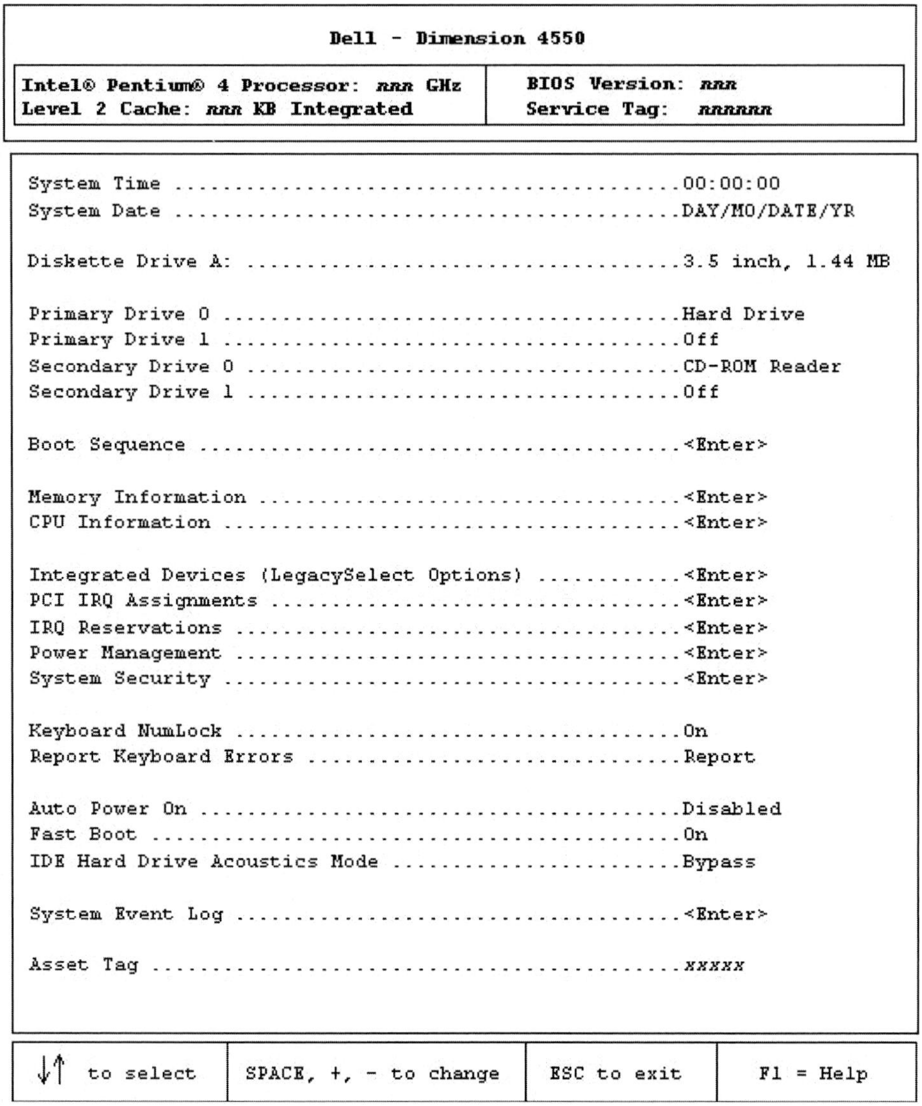

```
                        Dell - Dimension 4550

Intel® Pentium® 4 Processor: nnn GHz    BIOS Version: nnn
Level 2 Cache: nnn KB Integrated        Service Tag:  nnnnnn
```

```
System Time .........................................00:00:00
System Date .........................................DAY/MO/DATE/YR

Diskette Drive A: ...................................3.5 inch, 1.44 MB

Primary Drive 0 .....................................Hard Drive
Primary Drive 1 .....................................Off
Secondary Drive 0 ...................................CD-ROM Reader
Secondary Drive 1 ...................................Off

Boot Sequence .......................................<Enter>

Memory Information ..................................<Enter>
CPU Information .....................................<Enter>

Integrated Devices (LegacySelect Options) ..........<Enter>
PCI IRQ Assignments .................................<Enter>
IRQ Reservations ....................................<Enter>
Power Management ....................................<Enter>
System Security .....................................<Enter>

Keyboard NumLock ....................................On
Report Keyboard Errors ..............................Report

Auto Power On .......................................Disabled
Fast Boot ...........................................On
IDE Hard Drive Acoustics Mode .......................Bypass

System Event Log ....................................<Enter>

Asset Tag ...........................................xxxxx
```

```
↓↑  to select  |  SPACE, +, - to change  |  ESC to exit  |  F1 = Help
```

Figure 1-3
BIOS screenshot.

document perhaps) are both loaded into RAM from the hard drive at the beginning of an editing session. The *program* tells the CPU how to work on the *data*: in this case how to edit text. A *program instruction* would say something like "add the value in location X (*data*) to the value in location Y and update Y with the new value." For text

editing, the instructions might say "replace the letter 'a' in location X with the letter 'e'."

As in Fig. 1-4, the text paragraph (data) that is actively undergoing modification is held (in duplicate to the RAM copy) in the L2 cache, and the target sentence (in duplicate to the L2 copy) is manipulated from the L1 cache. Discrepancies

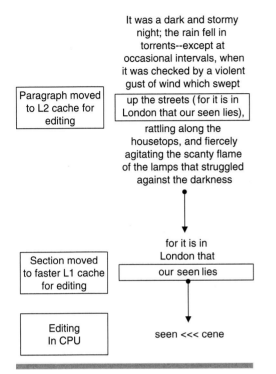

It was a dark and stormy night; the rain fell in torrents--except at occasional intervals, when it was checked by a violent gust of wind which swept

Paragraph moved to L2 cache for editing

up the streets (for it is in London that our seen lies),

rattling along the housetops, and fiercely agitating the scanty flame of the lamps that struggled against the darkness

for it is in London that

Section moved to faster L1 cache for editing

our seen lies

Editing In CPU

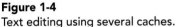

seen <<< cene

Figure 1-4
Text editing using several caches.

Table 1-1 Relative Speeds of Different Memory Types

Memory Type	Size	Access Speed
Processor	28 bytes	-10^9 times/s
L1 cache (SRAM)	32 KB	Same as processor
L2 cache (SRAM)	512 KB	1/2 L1 cache
Main memory (DRAM)	256 MB	1/6 L2 cache
Hard disk	Gigabytes	1/30 main memory

It is important to realize just how slow memory can be compared to the processor. Even the fastest hard disks have an access time measuring around 10 ms. If it has to wait 10 ms, a 200 MHz CPU will sit idle for 2 million clock cycles between each cycle devoted to useful work! And CD-ROMs are generally at least 10 times slower than hard disks. This is why using the much faster caches as holding pens (containing duplicates of information already stored elsewhere) is infinitely preferable to continuously accessing these much slower devices.

System Buses

All of the devices within a computer need to communicate with one another, and while there are wireless and optical approaches to data communication *between* computers, information is transferred by buses (which can be thought of as wires) *within* a computer.

There are a number of buses in a typical PC, the specifics of which are not as important as their general function. One major contributor to the speed of a computer is the width of its main buses, which have names like the system, backside, frontside, or I/O bus. A bus is a data path. Data travels along that path in parallel (like a rank of soldiers), with a group of data (such as the eight bits of a byte) traveling in unison from one point to another in the computer at intervals determined by the computer's clock. The width of the data path has a major impact on the overall speed of the computer, much as the number of lanes on a highway determines the amount of traffic it can handle concurrently. While older

among the duplicate copies are reconciled continuously. With modern memory architectures, which are very good at looking ahead, the processor will find the data element or program instruction it needs in one of the caches more than 90% of the time.

RAM (DRAM) consists of *single in-line memory modules* (SIMMs) or, more recently, in *dual in-line memory modules* (DIMMs). These are packaged on little circuit boards that are plugged into sockets on the motherboard (see Fig. 1-3). Consequently, RAM can be swapped out and upgraded in size or speed relatively easily. RAM costs have decreased dramatically over the past decade, at the same time (not coincidentally) that operating systems and other software have come to require more memory to perform efficiently. Finally, *virtual memory* is memory on the hard disk that is treated by the operating system as if it were really RAM (Table 1-1).

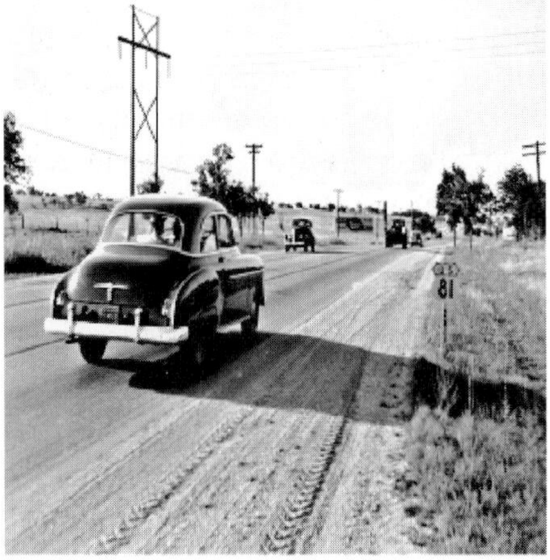

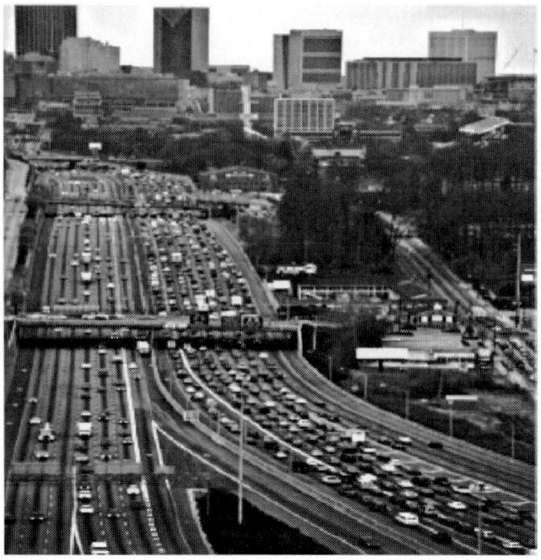

Compare traffic capacity of two lane road vs. multilane highway

Figure 1-5
Computer buses are like roads in that the amount of "traffic" they move is a function of the number of available channels.

computers had data paths of 8 bits (think 8 lanes), new Pentium class computers have 64 bit wide data paths (Fig. 1-5).

The width of the I/O bus, by which all peripherals (hard drive, CD-ROM, network card) communicate with the computer, also has a major impact on the computer's performance. The standards determining the architecture and speed of the I/O bus have generally evolved to keep pace with the increasing speed of the CPU. The original I/O bus was called, unimaginatively, the Industry Standard Architecture (ISA), and was 8 bits wide. This standard was extended, and became the extended ISA (EISA), which was faster. However, the EISA standard is now only of historical interest, having been replaced by the peripheral component interconnect (PCI) and the small computer systems interface (SCSI) bus standards, which are found on most new computers. The PCI bus is substantially faster than all prior standards and should be around for awhile. SCSI is a little more complicated in that it requires more customization for a specific computer, but it is fast and permits the attachment of multiple components to one bus (Table 1-2).

Table 1-2   Various Buses and Speeds

Bus Type	Bus Width	Bus Speed	Megabits/s
ISA	16 bits	8 MHz	16 MBps
EISA	32 bits	8 MHz	32 MBps
VL-bus	32 bits	25 MHz	100 MBps
VL-bus	32 bits	33 MHz	132 MBps
PCI	32 bits	33 MHz	132 MBps
PCI	64 bits	33 MHz	264 MBps
PCI	64 bits	66 MHz	512 MBps
PCI	64 bits	133 MHz	1 GBps
Synch SCSI	8 bits	5 MHz	5 MBps
Wide SCSI	16 bits	5 MHz	10 MBps
Fast SCSI	8 bits	10 MHz	10 MBps
Ultra SCSI	8 bits	20 MHz	20 MBps
Ultra3 SCSI	16 bits	40 MHz	160 MBps
USB 1.1	Serial	Not applicable	12 MBps
USB 2.0	Serial	Not applicable	480 MBps
Firewire (Apple)	Serial	Not applicable	400 MBps

The one major evolving computing function that *wasn't* accommodated by the PCI bus relates to the increasing demands of graphics intensive software, with 2 and 3D video consuming enormous amounts of bandwidth. This problem was solved with the development of an independent bus (like a private highway) dedicated solely to graphics traffic. The accelerated graphics port (AGP) sits physically at the intersection of several other buses, and is twice the speed of the PCI bus. Most new mid or upper level PCs are equipped with ISA, PCI, and AGP capabilities, permitting the concurrent use of legacy (older) ISA cards, PCI cards, and new high-end graphics cards, which use the AGP (see Fig. 1-6).

The universal serial bus (USB) and Apple's Firewire were developed to permit users to run peripheral devices without physically installing boards, allocating computer resources, configuring the devices, or powering the computer down every time a new piece of equipment (i.e., a camera) is attached. Up to 127 individual peripheral devices can be connected to a computer using USB ports. It is very simple to plug a USB device into the computer, because USB devices are automatically recognized and configured by the operating system. They can use power from the system or be connected to their own power supply.

The Central Processing Unit

The CPU has been left for last in this section, because it is both the most important component and the most difficult to describe. The CPU can be treated as a black box into which flow two channels: a data channel and an instruction channel. Inside the black box, the instructions determine what is done to the data, and the altered data flows out. The CPU's clock determines the speed with which these activities are executed.

Some of the issues relevant to discussions of the CPU include the manufacturer of the unit, its speed, and its instruction architecture. Intel is the name most people identify with processor

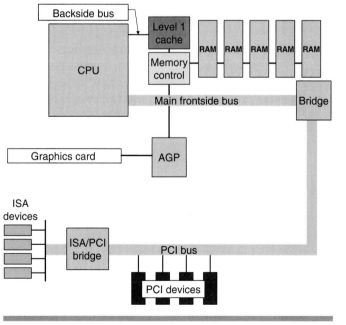

Figure 1-6
PC data bus map.

development, but it does have competitors, including Motorola (PowerPC) and Advanced Micro Devices (AMD) which have developed processors that outperform same-generation Intel's in price and/or performance.

The speed of a processor is a function of the width of its internal buses, the use of internal caching, its clock speed, and the accuracy with which it anticipates its next activity. While this last concept may seem obscure, a CPU has logic that attempts to enhance the efficiency of the computer by "predicting" what it will need to do next. Without going into detail, new processors use concepts described as *speculation, prediction,* and *explicit parallelism* to maximize the degree to which the CPU uses each tick of the clock (or clock cycle) for useful work.

Finally, two very different approaches to the implementation of instructions can be found in today's computers. The term instruction, in this case, refers to the fundamental computer directive that tells the processor what to do in each clock cycle. A "high level" language like Basic or C++ consists of commands representing sequences of these more basic ("low level") instructions. One approach or architecture is called a complex instruction set computer (CISC), in which there are a large variety of explicit instructions that may tell the computer

what to do for the next several cycles. The alternative approach, a reduced instruction set computer (RISC), uses a more limited number of simple instructions that execute very quickly, usually in one cycle. While there are advantages and disadvantages to each methodology, many of today's CPUs use instructions from both families to maximize performance.

Motherboard Summary

The motherboard has evolved in terms of its shape (known as its *footprint*) and its organization as rapid advances in CPU technology have compelled the development of clever ways in which to deliver data and instructions ever more rapidly. Gordon Moore, the cofounder of Intel, predicted in 1965 that the number of transistors on an integrated circuit would double every 18 months. While his eponymously named prediction (Moore's law) was originally forecast for 10 years, it has remained true for 35 and is expected to continue to be accurate until the middle of the second decade of this century (Fig. 1-7).

If the motherboard and its components represent the brain, central nervous system, and the protective endoskeleton of a computer, the organs are the power supply, the cooling fans, and the

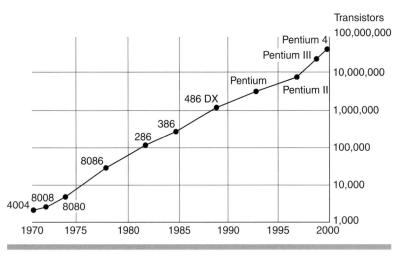

Figure 1-7
Moore's law.

devices found in most modern PCs, including storage devices, sound, and communication cards.

Motherboard Attachments

Key Points

- The power supply controls the electrical current to the computer.
- Memory storage can be permanently or removably attached to the motherboard, and include floppy drives, hard disk drives, CDs, DVDs, and flash drives.
- The network interface card (NIC) is the hardware through which the computer talks to the network and therefore other computers.
- Humans interact with the computer using input and output devices tailored for our senses (sight and sound) and appendages (hands).
- Evolving technologies (haptics, heads-up displays) based on the study of human-computer interface will refine the interactions between humans and computers.

The Computer Power Supply

The power supply is a hard-working, unglamorous part of all computers, in which alternating current is converted to direct current of various voltages, which is in turn used by the computer chips to power the transistors of which they are made. The power supply is attached in some way to all of the devices in the computer, including the motherboard, the drives, the expansion cards, and the fans.

Much as a biological heart can fail as additional load is placed on it, a computer's power supply may be insufficient to supply the correct voltage to the computer as optional devices are added into expansion slots. Alternatively, it may age and fail, eventually causing the PC to behave erratically.

The power supply is equipped with a fan which draws hot air out of the computer, cooling the inside, and thereby the CPU. The fan can wear out, often becoming noisy as it does so. When it stops working, the interior of the computer case can overheat, causing components to overheat and fail.

Long-Term (Non-RAM) Memory Storage Devices

The power supply has power attachments for the motherboard and devices like the floppy, CD-ROM, and hard drives. These devices are slower and cheaper memory storage devices than RAM, but are able to store enormous amounts of information.

True floppy disk drives, which are now archaic, were standardized at 5.25 in. and held 600 KB, or 1.2 MB on a "double density disk." The successor format is the 3.5 in. format, which holds 1.44 MB of data and is still found on most PCs. Today's internal hard disk drives have capacities of up to 100 GB. Both floppy and hard disk drives use the same method for data recording. They have one or more circular platters coated with ferromagnetic material. Data is inscribed by changing the polarity of a small region of the material on the disk. Disk "heads" move over the spinning disk and read or write information as necessary. A hard disk drive may have several disk platters and several heads (Fig. 1-8).

One major determinant of hard disk performance is the interface from the disk to the rest of the system, which uses one of the I/O buses. The disk itself can be quite fast but performance poor when data access is constrained by a slow bus, which acts as a choke point.

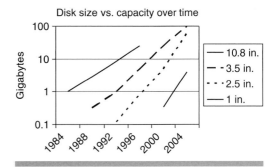

Figure 1-8
Affordable memory storage capacity has increased substantially over the past two decades.

The CD-ROM, once the standard for large removable storage disks, holds 600–700 MB of information. The major drawback to CDs in the past was the inability to write data to a CD. CD-ROMs are mass-produced and data are written once using tiny pits in the plastic surface of the disc (actually the lower surface, covered by a transparent upper surface). Newer CD-ROMs are writable disks and use colored dyes on the disk to encode data. They can be "burned" once by a user and subsequently reread many times. CD-RW disks contain phase-change material that can be written and overwritten repeatedly. The DVD, which is rapidly replacing the CD, has a much higher capacity and can be configured in formats ranging from 5 to 17 GB depending on whether one or two layers and one or two sides are used on the disk. Writable DVDs are also available in the DVD-R and DVD-RW formats.

The newest entry in the portable memory storage family is variously called a thumb drive, flash drive, USB drive, jump drive, keychain drive, or disk-on-key. It is a plug-and-play portable storage device that uses flash memory—the same kind of read-only memory used in the BIOS, as well as in camera memory cards. Flash memory does not have moving parts and is therefore noiseless and fast. A USB drive can be used in place of a floppy disk or CD, and when the user plugs the device into a USB port, the operating system recognizes it as a removable drive and assigns it a drive letter. Unlike most removable drives, a USB drive doesn't require rebooting, batteries, an external power supply, and is not operating system dependent. USB drives are available in capacities ranging from 8 MB to 2 GB.

The capacity numbers are meaningless in isolation, so it is useful to think of them in terms of real-world, tangible equivalents. One pulp-fiction mystery novel can be stored on less than 1 MB of hard disk storage, or on a floppy disk. One CD can contain over 1000 typical pulp novels and up to 10 times that number when data compression is used. The Encyclopedia Britannica can be stored on 1 GB of storage, which can also be used to store 1 hour of video.

Network Interface: NICs and Modems

Whereas the original PCs were invariably stand-alone devices, modern PCs are equipped with modems (*mo*dulation-*dem*odulation devices) and with NICs. Portable PCs are now equipped with wireless network interface hardware as well. The original application of a modem in the late 1980s and early 1990s was to access dial-up bulletin boards, on which one might find useful programs (such as software updates) or information. The demand for network interfaces of one sort or another (and dialing in to a network by modem is one approach), burgeoned with the rapid growth of the Internet and the development of business networks in the 1990s. There are any number of interfaces with various speeds, technologies, and symmetries (asymmetric interfaces permit faster communications in one direction than another). The relative speeds, technology, and other characteristics of currently available digital communications technologies are detailed in Table 1-3.

Regardless of the delivery medium, and it could be a phone line, cable modem, local area network, or even wireless transmission, network data (i.e., email, web pages) are ultimately delivered to a circuit board in the computer (typically the modem or a NIC). That board is responsible for decoding the information from its electronic format and delivering it to the PC. It is at the lowest level of what is called the protocol stack, that messages that have been broken up (and possibly encrypted) for delivery over a network such as the Internet are reconstructed. The network card or modem, like other devices, uses one of the I/O buses, such as the ISA or PCI bus, to interact with main memory and the CPU.

Human Computer Interface

The remaining components of a PC are the devices through which it communicates with the rest of the world. These include the video monitor, keyboard, mouse, joystick, speakers, microphone and more recently, camera. In effect, these technologies represent the voice and sense organs of a computer; and much as the sense organs of a human

Table 1-3   Various Computer Communication Technologies and Characteristics

Channel Type	Speed	Year	Description
TAT-1	51-calls	1956	The first transatlantic coaxial telephone cable, 7802 km out-of-service retired 1978
Dataphone	300bps	1958	1st modem: Bell Labs, Hayes AT commands
1,200 baud	1.2K	1962	2nd modem speed. Basic telephone line transmission rate
POTS	1.2K	1877	Plain old telephone service, the first commercial telephones
2,400 baud	2.4K	1980	3rd modem speed
Facsimile	9.6K	1980	FAX machines/FAX modems
9,600 baud	9.6K	1984	4th modem speed
14,400 baud	14.4K	1991	V.32bis modem, V.17 fax
28,800 baud	28.8K	1994	V.34, Rockwell V.Fast modems
33,600 baud	33.6K	1996	Maximum data transmission rate with copper telephone wires
N-ISDN	64.0K	1976	Narrowband integrated services digital network
GPRS	114.0K	1999	General packet radio service, RF in space (wireless)
UART 16650	460.8K	1995	Universal asynchronous receiver-transmitter, 32-byte buffer
UART 16750	921.6K	1995	Universal asynchronous receiver-transmitter, 64-byte buffer
T-1	1.544M	1957	Trunk level 1, 24 channels ($1 \times$ T1) time-division multiplexing by: AT&T
ISDN-PRI	1.544M	1988	Primary rate interface $23 \times 64K$ B-channels, $1 \times 64K$ D-channel on T1, 23B + D
IrDA	4.000M	1994	Infrared data association, wireless communication standard
10Base-T	10.000M	1995	100 m, Ethernet (unshielded twisted pair) Cat3
Standard SCSI	10.000M	1995	SCSI-1, small computer system interface
USB 1.1	12.000M	1996	5 m, universal serial bus, external bus standard
Token ring	16.000M	1982	LAN, a type of computer network by: IBM
Ultra SCSI	40.000M	1993	SCSI-3, small computer system interface
T-3	44.736M	1991	Trunk level 3, 672 channels ($28 \times$ T1) time-division multiplexing by: AT&T
AGP 2.0	266.000M	1998	Accelerated graphics port by: Intel
Firewire	400.000M	1995	A serial SCSI variant developed by Apple
USB 2.0	480.000M	1999	Universal serial bus, external bus standard v2.0
TAT-9	565.000M	1991	Fiberoptic cable network laid from North America to Europe
SONET	2.488G	1988	Synchronous Optical NETwork-Designed by the Telcos
FLAG	5.300G	1997	Fiberoptic link around the globe, 27,300 km linking Great Britain and Japan

are optimized to communicate information about our particular environment, the computer's interface devices are optimized for communication with a human (Fig. 1-9).

This is not to say that other forms of interfaces haven't been designed. A NIC or modem, for example, is designed for computer communication with a network. Other nonhuman interface sensors are designed to detect mechanical (e.g., automobile computers) or biological behavior and communicate that information to the computer.

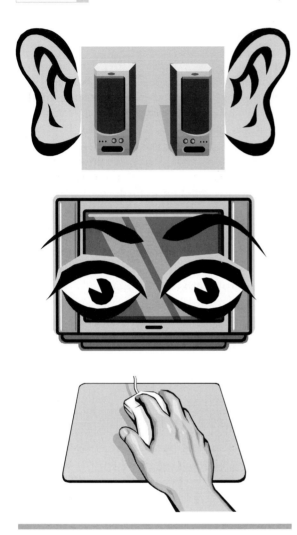

Figure 1-9
Computer input and output devices are designed to "interface" with human eyes, ears, and hands—futurists have described direct interfaces with the human mind.

Video Cards and Monitors

Early PCs featured a black and white or black and amber monochrome monitor, and designed for text rendering. The evolution of windowed (graphically oriented) operating systems (from Apple and Microsoft) spurred the development of higher resolution monitors and sophisticated graphics cards, which in turn permitted the development of 2D

computer games. Some of the graphics standards that have been widely implemented are shown in Table 1-4.

The graphics capabilities of low-end PCs have converged with those of computer assisted design (CAD) computers, which were designed for sophisticated architectural and engineering rendering during the early 1990s. Today's graphics cards, which include hardware dedicated to 3D and texture rendering, are a product of that convergence and, more recently, the consumer demands of the gaming market.

Computer games such as Doom, Myst, Quake, and others have very sophisticated visual (and sound) landscapes, and feature rapid, realistic image rendering as the player's viewpoint changes. The implementation of the AGP (as described above), the inclusion of special video memory on video boards, and the development of very fast graphics hardware have revolutionized computer video displays. Video technology now permits the display of 2 megapixels (1600 × 1200 pixel displays) in 16 million colors, and resolutions of 10–15 mega pixels are on the horizon.

Advances in monitor technology have paralleled advances in image rendering hardware. While the

Table 1-4

Computer Resolution Standards	Designation Resolution (in Pixels)	Total Pixels on the Screen
VGA (video graphics array)	640 × 480	300 kilo pixels (KP)
SVGA (super VGA)	800 × 600	480 KP
XGA (extended graphics array)	1024 × 768	790 KP
SXGA (super XGA)	1280 × 1024	1.3 megapixels (MP)
UXGA (ultra XGA)	1600 × 1200	1.9 MP
QXGA (quad XGA)	2048 × 1536	3.1 MP
QSXGA	2560 × 2048	5.2 MP
QUXGA	3200 × 2400	7.7 MP
HSXGA (hexadecimal SXGA)	5120 × 4096	21 MP
HUXGA	6400 × 4800	31 MP

cathode ray tube (CRT) has been the historical standard for image display, new technologies such as liquid crystal displays (LCDs) and, now, the gas plasma screen will increasingly predominate (Fig. 1-10).

The principles of the CRT, wherein an electron gun is aimed at light-emitting (emissive), colored phosphors on a screen, are well understood. The technology is mature and relatively inexpensive. Its downsides are the size and weight of the CRT, its energy consumption, and the emission of electromagnetic radiation. LCD displays have evolved rapidly, driven in part by the laptop computer market. LCDs display images by filtering light emitted by a backlight behind the screen. The technology is therefore described as *transmissive*. Color is generated by using three cells (red, green, and blue) per pixel, wherein the ultimate color of the viewed pixel is determined by the relative transmission of each cell in the pixel. The terms passive and active matrix have been applied to color LCDs. The former indicates a less expensive, less bright, less sharp display than the latter.

The latest flat panel displays are *emissive* and phosphor based like CRTs, but like LCDs in that they consist of grids of electrodes in the screen. Plasma display panels (PDPs) can be thought of as matrices of pixels with red, green, and blue emissive phosphors in each of three subcells. PDPs are relatively inexpensive to produce, but have a limited lifespan and the technology man" therefore not suited to desktop displays and are more appropriate for large screen displays, as with high definition television or wall-mounted displays.

Rapid developments in flat-panel display will inevitably change the use of wall space in the home and workplace. Immersive environments, in which a computer controls wall displays and sound, have already been developed and are used in research, industrial design, scientific visualization, and gaming. These applications will become commonplace in clinical medicine in the near future. Obvious projects include the development of large, multipurpose, flat-panel displays that permit concurrent display of radiographic information in 2 or 3 dimensions, text and trended laboratory or physiologic data rendered using data visualization techniques. One can imagine displays of this sort replacing the unwieldy charts and binders we currently use.

Computer Sound

Speakers and sound cards are packaged with most new computers and, as with video, computer generated sound has become increasingly realistic and computationally intensive. While PCs were originally conceived of as business machines, capable only of rudimentary clicks and beeps, the advent of multimedia applications has spawned the development of increasingly sophisticated sound generation and recording software and hardware.

Programmers can now write software that characterizes an environment (e.g., concert hall) and the behavior of a sound (e.g., gunshot) in that environment, using standards such as the environmental audio extensions (EAX) developed by Creative Labs (the manufacturers of SoundBlaster cards). Another major impetus for the development of computer sound has been the development and maturation of the musical instrument digital interface (MIDI) interface, which has evolved to a general set of standards for computer music for controlling devices, such as synthesizers and sound cards that emit music. At minimum, a MIDI representation of a sound includes values for a note's pitch, length, and volume.

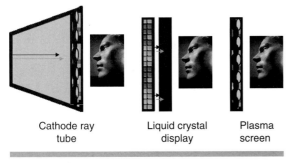

Cathode ray tube   Liquid crystal display   Plasma screen

Figure 1-10
The three prevalent display technologies use different approaches in creating color images.

The sounds of a large variety of musical instruments are characterized in MIDI (Fig. 1-11), and most synthesizers support the MIDI standard, so sounds created on one synthesizer can be played and manipulated on another. Computers with a MIDI interface can record sounds created by a synthesizer and then manipulate the data to produce new sounds. For example, the key of a stretch of music can be changed with a single keystroke.

Perhaps the best testament to the growing importance of computer sound is the fact that the MIDI standards described above are hard-wired into sound chips integrated into many of the newer motherboards, rather than necessitating a separate add-on ISA or PCI board. One can expect that hardware for the optimization of computer-synthesized speech will be commonplace in the next few years.

Input Devices (Keyboards, Mice, Microphones, Cameras)

A personal computer would only be an interesting piece of electronic statuary if it lacked some way for humans to communicate with it. The options

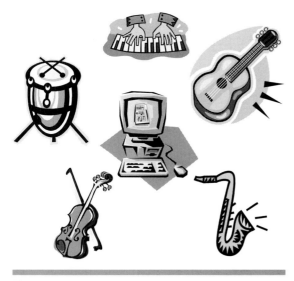

Figure 1-11
MIDI is the computer standard used by computers to encode music and the sounds of instruments.

for human to computer (as contrasted with computer to human) interaction increase every day and there is an evolving science studying human computer interaction (HCI).

Haptics is one area of HCI, and is the science of applying touch sensation and control to interaction with computer applications. Using special I/O devices (joysticks, data gloves, or other devices), computer users can get tactile feedback from computer applications in the form of sensations in the hand or other parts of the body. There are a number of extreme useful applications of haptics. When combined with a visual display, haptics can be used to train people for tasks requiring hand-eye coordination, such as surgery or remote object manipulation. Haptics can also be used for games providing virtual feedback in interactions with virtual objects. For example, one might play tennis with another gamer somewhere on the Internet; and both players can see the moving ball, position and swing the haptic tennis racket, and feel the impact of the ball.

Where keyboards were the only input options with the first, text-oriented PCs, windowed operating systems (Windows, Apple) led to the development of a mouse for efficient interaction with the window contents. Microphones, video cameras, joysticks, and gloves are among the growing number of additional devices that are now in common use as input devices. Joysticks and gloves are widely available, and haptic versions of each are becoming commercially available (e.g. the Microsoft Sidewinder joystick) (Fig. 1-12).

Biometrics and computer vision is another increasingly important application of HCI. Biometrics is the measurement of unique human characteristics (such as facial geometry, retinal vascular patterns, iris patterns) to distinguish humans from one another for security purposes. Speech recognition is a developing, sound-oriented application of HCI (Fig. 1-13).

▮ Summary

The capabilities of PCs are growing exponentially, as is the speed. Intranets, the Internet and the Next Generation Internet provide the capability for

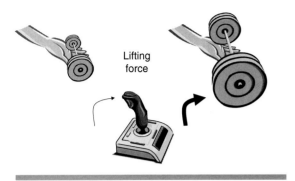

Figure 1-12
Haptic devices give tactile feedback to the user as, for example, the force needed to manipulate a virtual weight.

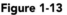

Figure 1-13
Fingerprints can be used for biometric identification using a biometric touchpad on a mouse: (a) digital fingerprint is acquired from which, (b) a template is made, and (c) the template is matched to the user of a biometrically enabled mouse to authenticate the user.

intercomputer communication with the potential for unimaginable synergies. One group, for example, was able to decipher a supposedly secure encryption scheme using time simultaneously donated by tens of thousands of computers (that would otherwise have been sitting idle at the time).

Many of the current routine applications of computers in medicine are relatively mundane; but as their capabilities grow, we can expect to see ever more interaction between health care providers and "smart" computers. This chapter is intended to provide the reader with an understanding of how computers function, their fundamental anatomy, and the implications of their growing capabilities for medical care.

Suggested Readings

Gilster R. *PC Hardware: A Beginner's Guide*. McGraw-Hill: Berkeley, Osborne, 2001.

White R, Downs TE. *How Computers Work*, 7th ed. Indianapolis, Que, 2001.

2

Software

Operating System: Introduction

The operating system can be thought of as the government of a computer. Unlike the hardware circuitry, which is inherently fixed, like governments, the operating system can be structured in a variety of ways. Each of the Windows families, the Macintosh family and Linux are operating systems that can run on essentially the same set of circuitry.

Operating systems were originally designed to run on large mainframes, where they had essentially the same function as they do on today's personal computers and laptops. However, many of today's handheld devices, such as personal digital assistants and cell phones, also have operating systems. In fact, the computer in a modern cell phone is more powerful than that of a 20-year-old desktop personal computer. It is possible for computers to run without an operating system, and the computers that control most household appliance are hard-wired, self-contained computers designed to perform one set of tasks very efficiently. While this is obviously attractive, it is inflexible, doesn't permit the application of updates, patches, fixes, and therefore condemns a computing device to slow obsolescence. It is entirely possible and some sophisticated users choose to install two different operating systems on the same computer. In this case, the user can choose to "boot" into one or the other system at the time of booting up the computer. The operating system is the first thing that is loaded onto a computer in a process called bootstrapping, which will be described below, and without it, the computer cannot work.

Bootstrapping and BIOS

Key Points

- Power-on self-test (POST) for hardware components in the system to make sure everything is working properly.
- Activating other basic input-output system (BIOS) chips on cards installed in the computer, i.e., SCSI and graphics cards.
- Provides low-level routines used by the operating system to interface to different input, output, and other hardware devices, i.e., the keyboard, the screen, and the serial and parallel ports.
- Manage settings for the hard disks, clock, and so on.

Computer Power On

The first thing that happens when a computer is turned on is an activity wherein a set of instructions called the BIOS are run from the computer's read-only memory (ROM). The BIOS loads interrupt handlers and device drivers and it initializes the computer's registers and power management. Interrupt handlers are small programs acting as translators between hardware components, like the mouse and keyboard, and the operating system. When the user presses a key on the keyboard, the value or name of that key is stored in a buffer (temporary storage area) and the keyboard sends an interrupt to the operating system indicating that there is something in the buffer. The operating system can decide what to do about the interrupt and when. Some keyboard combinations (like Ctrl, Alt, Delete pressed together) may generate interrupts that have a higher priority than others and therefore get attention sooner. Device drivers are pieces of code that identify the base hardware components and their features for the operating system.

Power-On Self-Test

The next piece of business for the BIOS is a program called the POST, by which the computer takes stock of itself and key components like the CPU, main memory (RAM), and BIOS. Following a successful test, the several device drivers are activated. One of the device drivers handles the video card, which the BIOS activates early in its sequence (Fig. 2-1). This driver turns on the display and the user can "watch" the rest of the boot-up sequence culminating in the logon prompt from the operating system. The video card may have its own BIOS to initialize the memory and graphics-processing unit on the card. Once the video card is active the BIOS moves on to turn on other cards on the motherboard, such as personal computer interface and small computer system interface cards. Details about these devices are displayed on the video screen as each of them are identified and characterized.

Bootstrapping

Finally, the BIOS activates the computer's disk drives and looks for the operating system's base or start-up program, the *bootstrap loader*. This program has a single function, which is to load the operating system into memory. The bootstrap loader checks the disk drives (hard drives, floppy drives, and CD drives) in a specific sequence looking for the operating system. The message "non-system disk or disk error," often encountered when floppy drives were in common use indicated that the operating system found a disk in the floppy drive that was not a "system" (as in operating system) disk.

The BIOS may need periodic updating, which is not a job for the faint of heart. BIOS's can be downloaded and installed from computer manufacturer's web sites, but it takes an experienced user to perform the task since failure to get it right

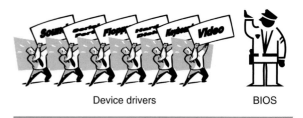

Figure 2-1
The BIOS "loads" the drivers for all of the devices used by a computer.

can paralyzed a computer. BIOS updates were necessary, for example, to allow PCs to handle the date issue during the Y2K transition.

What is an OS?

The intent of an operating system is to have a reliable and consistent method by which to organize and control hardware and software from session to session and moment to moment. In order to be called an operating system, a body of software should be expected to perform a specific set of jobs. The OS manages the hardware and software assets of the system including the central processing unit, memory, disk space, interface devices, and so on. It should also provide a consistent, stable exterior or "shell" with which applications and the people who program them can expect to interact.

If the choice of a specific operating system, be it Windows, Macintosh, or Linux, is like the choice of a style of government, the actual management of the hardware and software assets of a computer is analogous to the management of the infrastructure of a city. A number of different resources need to be managed in synchrony for optimal efficiency of the overall system. Programs require processing time, specific elements from memory, interaction with the user through the keyboard and/or mouse, and all that in an orchestrated fashion so for example, the wrong memory element doesn't arrive at the wrong time or too late. In addition, several programs run concurrently in most modern personal computers, making the orchestration task infinitely more complex. These jobs are the core work-product of an operating system. The other key feature of today's operating systems is their ability (or the lack thereof) to function consistently across a variety of "platforms", meaning the hardware elements of a PC including the speed of its processor, the amount of on-board memory, and its components.

Operating System Architectures

Key Points

- A real-time operating system (RTOS) is solely dedicated to doing one task.
- Single-user, single task operating systems are used on cell phones and personal digital assistants.
- Single-user, multitasking operating systems run personal computers.
- Multiuser, multitasking operating systems are found on mainframe computers.

Operating systems actually come in one of four categories (Fig. 2-2). A common but little known variety is what is called a RTOS, used to control machinery, scientific instruments, and industrial systems. A RTOS usually lacks a user interface capability and functions as an embedded system. Its job is usually to ensure that a required operation occurs on time and in a specific, predictable amount of time *every* time. Functions occurring too early (such as the movement of a robot arm) or too late can have catastrophic consequences.

Single-user, single task operating systems are designed to manage operations wherein a sole user does one task at a time. Cell phones and personal digital assistants fit this description as did the original PCs prior to the advent of windowed operating systems.

Single-user multitasking describes most of today's personal computers and the function of the operating systems on them. While there are a variety of subtleties to the meaning of multitasking, the principle is that the user can functionally run a number of programs concurrently, such as reading email while downloading a file from a web site and writing a document on a word processor. In reality, the central processing unit

Real time OS: Single user/single
no human user   process OS

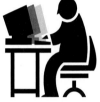

Single user/multi-   Multi-user/multi-
process OS   process OS

Figure 2-2
There are several different categories of operating systems.

is cycling among these jobs, but the cycling occurs so quickly that they appear to be happening at the same time.

Finally, mainframe computers service many users simultaneously and are therefore multiuser, multitasking devices. Historically, this was the only kind of computer available and users interacted with them using "dumb" terminals, which were keyboard and video screens. Today's users are much more likely to interact with a mainframe through their PC, as a scientific user might "upload" a computationally intensive task from a PC to a mainframe.

Operating System Tasks

Key Points

- Processor management—Break tasks down into manageable chunks and prioritizing them before assignment to the CPU.
- Memory management—Coordinate the flow of data in and out of RAM and determine when to use virtual memory.

- Storage management—Direct where data will be stored.
- Device management—Providing an interface among each device, the CPU, and applications which need the devices.
- Application interface—Provide for communications and data exchange between software applications and the computer.
- User interface—Provide a way for the user to interact with the computer.

The operating system has six general tasks: processor management, memory management, storage management, device management, management of the applications interface, and the user interface. Processor management implies the efficient use of the main engine of the computer, i.e., making sure that each of the applications running at a given time can run fast enough to function properly and that the CPU is doing something useful as much of the time as possible.

Process Management

Operating systems deal in processes (or threads depending on the operating system), which are organized computing activities that may or may not have a 1:1 relationship to an application (such as a word processing program). A process or thread might be dedicated to communication among programs, virus scanning or memory network management, and the operating system needs to comanage their different and often competing needs. In general, then, the operating system distributes time among the various processes or threads according to their needs and priority. While this job is relatively simple in a single-user, single task environment, it becomes much more complicated in today's single user, multitasking environment, where any number of applications can be running concurrently and competing for the attention of the operating system (Fig. 2-3).

The way in which active processes coexist is as follows. Each process takes up residence in a certain

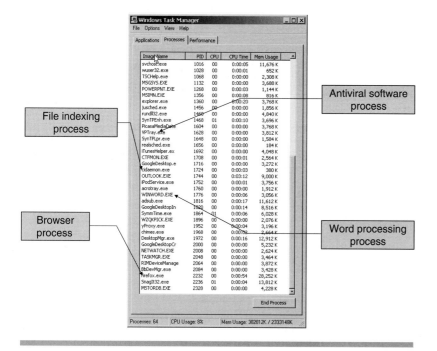

Figure 2-3
Personal computers run many processes concurrently.

amount of RAM. The operating system rotates central processor activity (cycles) among the active processes. When one process is due to take its turn, the OS loads the necessary information into central temporary storage locations called registers, stacks, and queues and then proceeds to work. This information typically includes a combination of data and instructions. When the process has used up its allotted time, the operating system copies the information from all of those temporary storage locations and stores it with a placeholder indicating where the work stopped somewhere in RAM. The OS then loads a second process into the same registers, stacks, and queues and gives it some processing time. While all of this is going on, the OS may be handling interrupt requests from other processes or hardware components.

Memory Management

The second major job of the operating system relates to memory management. As with management of the central processing unit, the OS must ensure that each process has enough memory to execute without interfering with another process. Additionally, given the fact that there are several types of memory (ranging from fast cache to disk space), the operating system should ensure that processes use memory optimally. The various types of memory are described in Chap. 1. One example of the kind of memory management and operating system might perform is the "reservation" of a chunk of disk memory to act as what is known as virtual memory—memory that appears to be located in random access memory (RAM) but is actually on a disk drive. In a sense, virtual memory is analogous to an overflow parking lot: it is preferable (more efficient) for a car (process) to park in the main parking lot, but parking in an overflow lot (read virtual memory) is better than parking in an off-site location and busing to the airport (Fig. 2-4).

Storage Management

Storage management is closely related to memory management and refers to the operating system's responsibility for longer-term storage of data and programs. Memory management is analogous to traffic direction and short-term parking, whereas storage management is more like long-term parking. For example, if a user wishes to work on a stored document, the operating system has to go to its storage location (on a hard disk or network drive), get it, get the program that will be used to edit it and feed them both into RAM and the caches.

Device Management

A third responsibility of the OS is device management. The conduit between every piece of hardware and the OS is a piece of software called a device driver, which acts as a translator between the pulses of electricity that the hardware knows about and the software or code that the operating system knows about. The flow of information goes in both directions through the conduit. A printer driver, for example, takes the output from a word processing program and tells the printer where to spray ink on a piece of paper to make the output document (Fig. 2-5). Similarly, a mouse driver takes input from the movement of the ball inside a mouse. The excursion of the ball indicates how far the mouse has moved in a vertical and horizontal direction, which is relayed to the operating system which, in turn, guides the cursor on the screen accordingly. Drivers are appended to an operating system rather than built in so that new hardware can be added to a computer, and packaged with a driver, without overhauling the OS (Fig. 2-6).

Applications Interface

The hardware of PC's vary substantially in terms of their internal architecture ranging from what central processor is used, what buses are available, to what devices (i.e., keyboard, mouse, video, disk drive, and so on) are installed. Today's user expects the operating system to "know about," recognize and interact efficiently with, all of these elements without the user's intervention. New operating systems typically allow the user to plug in a new device, and "play" it immediately: the so-called

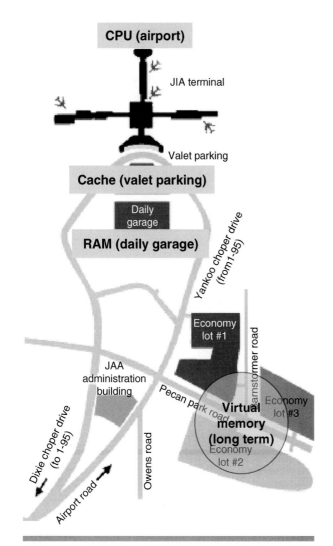

Figure 2-4
Computer memory is analogous to traffic management at an airport, where the terminal is the center of the action and is serviced by several levels of parking service ranging from valet (like cache memory) to long term (like virtual memory).

"plug and play" capability. Parenthetically, and as many of the readers will remember, operating systems of a decade ago, such as Windows 95, required a substantial amount of start-up and on-going maintenance to run and keep running. Today's operating systems are designed to know about how to function in a tremendous number of computer configurations; and when they don't recognize a piece of equipment, they have an idea about how to go about finding the desired information on the Internet.

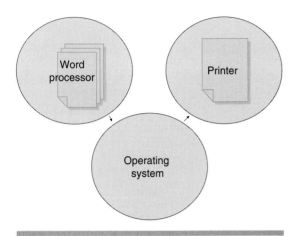

Figure 2-5
The operating system takes output from the word processing program and "queues" it for the printer.

Much of this flexibility is the result of consistent application program interfaces (APIs).

Understanding an API is critical to an understanding of what an OS does. A useful analogy is that of an electrical socket. All electrical devices wishing to use AC (alternating current) in the United States are equipped with plugs (which amount to interface devices) meeting certain specifications in terms of number, size, and distance between prongs. Furthermore, the electricity

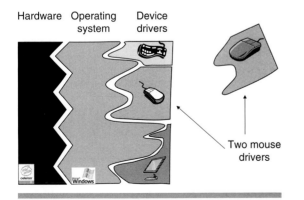

Figure 2-6
Device drivers interface with the operating system which, in turn, controls the hardware.

coming through the plug comes in the form of alternating rather than direct current, which has implications for the way in which the device uses the electricity. The plug itself and the electricity that comes through it conform to universal standards that a device can expect to find at every plug. The device doesn't care whether the electricity was originally formed by nuclear, hydraulic, or some other form of power generation. Bear in mind that there are other plug paradigms such the ones found in various places outside of the United States, where the prong specifications and current are quite different.

An API then is a consistent programmer's interface to the operating system through which a program can request certain services. For example, a program (such as a browser) may wish to open a new window on the screen. The browser program can ask the OS to "draw" a window of a certain size in a certain location using a "window API".

The beauty of this arrangement, in which the innards of the subprogram that draws the window are opaque to the program requesting the service, is that component programs (i.e., the window drawing program) can be swapped out and updated without any harm to the overall function of the system. There could be a variety of reasons that the window drawing program might need to be changed, including the development of more efficient approaches or remedies for security flaws in the old approach. In general, then, APIs represent predictable, consistent points and methods of attachment for programs wishing to do business with the OS.

In effect, the OS provides a set of widely used "attachment points" by which applications programmers can get work done by the OS. For example, it is very common for an application to create, open, and manipulate files. The OS provides a number of file management utilities by which an application can create, open, save, move, copy files. The operating system has the responsibility of making sure those instructions are handled efficiently and correctly on the computer hardware it is managing

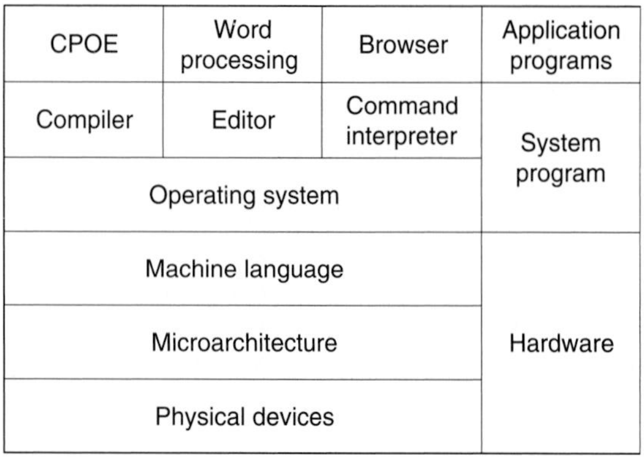

CPOE	Word processing	Browser	Application programs
Compiler	Editor	Command interpreter	System program
Operating system			
Machine language			Hardware
Microarchitecture			
Physical devices			

Figure 2-7
This schematic explicitly shows the layers of hardware and software and how they interact.

(Fig. 2-7). In other words, the application can use the same instructions with a given operating system whether the OS is installed on IBM, Dell, or Gateway hardware, all of which may be configured differently. Another twist on the API issue is that while some OSs are "open source," ones in which the code "behind" the operating system is available to programmers for inspection, such as Linux, or "closed" source, where the OS software is hidden from the applications programmer. Much of the Windows family code fits the latter description. The issues relating to open- and closed-source code will be discussed at greater length at the end of the chapter.

User Interface

The sixth and most visible job of an operating system is to interact with the user. Historically, computers interacted with users using a command line interface, wherein the user typed in a series of letters to initiate action on the part of the computer. The user interfaces in today's computers are graphical, as with Apple and Windows systems as well as the Linux operating system, which is typically bundled with two different graphical user interfaces (GUIs). All of these systems also provide an old fashioned command line

interface for direct interaction with the operating system. The Windows version is invoked by the Start/Run/Cmd sequence as seen below. The GUIs are a layer of software riding on top of the operating system (Fig. 2-8).

◼ Standard Operating System Utilities

Operating systems typically come with a variety of standard utilities allowing the user to manage files, security, system date and time, certain parameters about memory management (such as the size of virtual memory and disk partitioning), and task scheduling. Network management tools including personal firewalls are increasingly integrated into the operating system as well.

File Management Utilities

File management utilities allow the user to gather information about a file, such as its size and type. The filename was constrained to a limited number of characters in some of the early Windows versions, so that users were forced to work with names that were poorly descriptive of the file's contents. Other operating systems (such as Apple's) and newer versions of windows give the user a greater degree of latitude in the description of a file, although certain characters (such as dashes) cannot be used in the filename.

The use of the "filename.extension" paradigm dates back to mainframe computing, where a three-character extension was used to indicate to the operating system what the format of the file was. There were a relatively limited number of possible file formats, such as executable (".exe"), binary (".bin"), text (".txt"). The extension "told" the OS how to interpret the string of bits that any given file was made of. This is still the case in modern personal computers. If, for example, the user changes the extension of a file it will most likely become uninterpretable. For example, if one were to change the extension of a picture file from ".jpg," one of the standard picture formats to ".txt," a drawing program will not interpret the file properly and open it as a picture (Fig. 2-9).

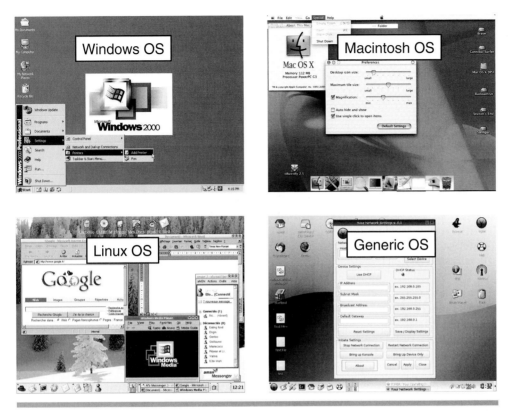

Figure 2-8
The graphical user interfaces (GUIs) of several operating systems.

Local Name	Size	Type	Modified	Remote Name	Size	Type	Modified	Attribute
My Documents		System Folder	05/10/2005 08:24:4...	3GENERATIONS MPEG-1.M...	50,765,456	Movie Clip	08/18/2000 02:18:2...	-rw-rw-r--
My Computer		System Folder		Artificial Intelligence.ppt	177,152	Microsoft PowerPoint Presentation	04/13/2004 09:04:5...	-rw-rw-r--
My Network Places		System Folder		asgn.html	4,886	HTML File	01/13/2005 02:57:0...	-rw-rw-r--
Recycle Bin		System Folder		assignments.html	964	HTML File	12/13/2001 03:00:3...	-rw-rw-r--
Internet Explorer		System Folder		astonbu1.gif	326	GIF Image	01/13/2005 02:25:0...	-rw-rw-r--
Ad-Aware SE Personal	682	Shortcut	01/25/2005 05:47:0...	astonbu2.gif	258	GIF Image	01/13/2005 02:25:0...	-rw-rw-r--
Adobe Acrobat 6.0 Professio...	1,559	Shortcut	09/23/2004 03:07:1...	astonbu3.gif	233	GIF Image	01/13/2005 02:25:0...	-rw-rw-r--
Adobe Reader 6.0	1,557	Shortcut	08/05/2004 01:46:0...	astonrul.gif	990	GIF Image	01/13/2005 02:25:0...	-rw-rw-r--
Grokker 2.1	652	Shortcut	05/20/2004 02:08:0...	Bioinformatics and Medicine....	546,304	Microsoft PowerPoint Presentation	04/15/2004 10:54:2...	-rw-rw-r--
Microsoft Baseline Security A...	729	Shortcut	05/20/2005 08:56:4...	Biosensors and Telerobotics....	196,065	Adobe Acrobat Document	04/17/2003 05:13:4...	-rw-rw-r--
Mozilla Firefox	1,491	Shortcut	05/16/2005 08:33:2...	Biosensors and Telerobotics....	55,808	Microsoft PowerPoint Presentation	04/14/2003 05:13:2...	-rw-rw-r--
Registry Mechanic	625	Shortcut	09/26/2004 09:59:2...	Celene Chang.ppt	2,777,088	Microsoft PowerPoint Presentation	04/12/2004 10:55:0...	-rw-rw-r--
SnagIt 7	1,598	Shortcut	05/28/2005 11:14:2...	Challenger Visualization.pdf	3,229,831	Adobe Acrobat Document	02/05/2003 03:45:1...	-rw-rw-r--
SSH Secure File Transfer Cli...	1,776	Shortcut	02/23/2005 10:00:3...	Challenger Visualization.ppt	8,855,552	Microsoft PowerPoint Presentation	02/04/2004 04:50:0...	-rw-rw-r--
SSH Secure Shell Client	830	Shortcut	02/23/2005 10:00:3...	CHpresentation.ppt	103,936	Microsoft PowerPoint Presentation	04/15/2004 04:10:5...	-rw-rw-r--
WinZip	625	Shortcut	02/04/2005 03:26:2...	CML.pdf	127,003	Adobe Acrobat Document	04/08/2003 02:03:2...	-rw-rw-r--

Figure 2-9
A typical file management utility showing files, their location, size, type, and date of most recent modification.

There are thousands of file formats in today's world of rapidly proliferating software, but the basic premise is that the operating system associates a given file extension with the file's function or the software with which it is associated.

A variety of dates and times are also associated with files including the date of creation, the date of most recent access, the date of most recent alteration. This information can be determined for a given file in several ways. Many programs, such as the word processing program with which this chapter is written, will display the properties of a file on request. Alternatively, the file management utility built into most operating systems (i.e., the Explorer utility in Windows or Macintosh operating systems) can provide a wealth of information about individual files.

Another key piece of information about a file's properties relates to its attributes and permissions. A file can be labeled "read only," meaning that it is protected from accidental or intentional modification or erasure. "Hidden" files are not visible unless the user knows the name of the file; critical operating system files may be labeled as "hidden" so as to protect them from inadvertent alteration by the user. Unfortunately, hackers may "hide" malicious files on a user's hard drive for more nefarious reasons. "Compression" is a process by which a file is evaluated and redundant or unused bits, analogous to the empty, white space on this page, are eliminated. Unix-based operating systems assign the right to "read," "write," and "execute" independently to the owner, a specific group of users or the public (Fig. 2-10).

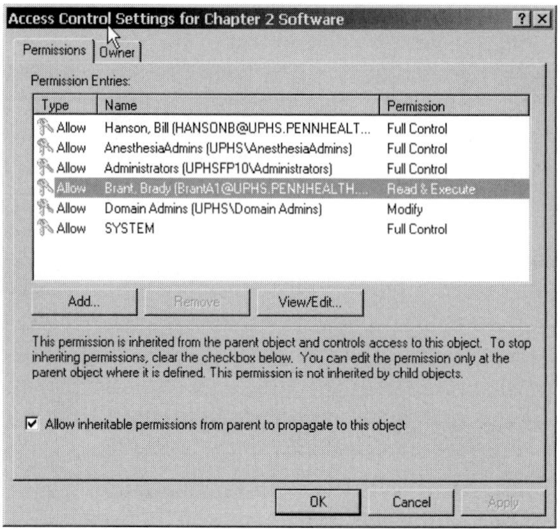

There are a variety of other attributes that are specific to a given operating or file management system. Novell Netware, for example, controls attributes pertaining to the right to modify a file's name and whether and when a file can be archived (stored to another storage device). Windows XP provides for permissions such as "write attributes."

Disk and User Management Utilities

It is increasingly important in modern operating systems to have the ability to control the privileges of multiple users on a single PC. The personal

Figure 2-10
The access permissions for a given file can be specified and relate to who can do what to that file.

computers found around a hospital, for example, are typically unsecured and accessible by a variety of health care workers. While a default user may be permitted to run certain applications and interact with the Internet, an "administrator" has additional rights. Similarly, an enterprise such as a hospital system may provide hardware and software to its employees but restrict their ability to customize its configuration. By so doing, the health system can ensure the legality (legal as opposed to pirated software) and interoperability (same versions of software) of the systems (Figs. 2-11 and 2-12).

A user may not be permitted to install new pieces of software such as operating system updates. Those functions are restricted to someone with administrative privileges. Similarly, a standard user may not be permitted to run a disk defragmentation (see below) program, a function constrained to "administrators." It is in the interests of the owners of computers in a corporate environment, such as a hospital, to control what software is installed on its machines and how they are operated. The operating system may also permit administrators to remotely control a

Name	Description
Administrators	Administrators have complete and unrestricted access to the computer/domain
Backup Operators	Backup Operators can override security restrictions for the sole purpose of backing up ...
Guests	Guests have the same access as members of the Users group by default, except for th...
Power Users	Power Users possess most administrative powers with some restrictions. Thus, Power ...
Replicator	Supports file replication in a domain
Users	Users are prevented from making accidental or intentional system-wide changes. Thus...
Debugger Users	Debugger users can debug processes on this machine, both locally and remotely
Remote Control Operators	

Figure 2-11
An operating system typically has a variety of generic access levels controlling the degree to which a user can control or modify the settings of the computer.

computer in order to allow for off-site troubleshooting and diagnostics.

Disk Maintenance

Disk management and maintenance are important to computer hygiene. In computers files are broken down into smaller pieces for storage on a hard or floppy disk. The disk has standard-sized "sectors," consisting of uniform stretches of magnetic recording material laid out according to the *formatting* rules of a given operating system.

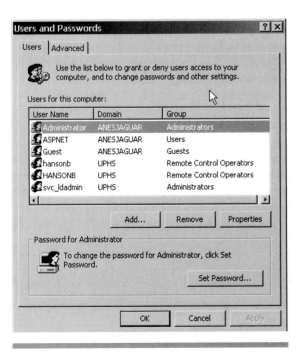

One way of thinking about this is that the unformatted disk is like an unlined playing field. Much as an athletic director may choose to line a field for soccer or football, an operating system chooses how to format a disk drive. Files stored on that disk drive must conform to its formatting layout. A newly created file, such as a text file, is stored in an unoccupied stretch of sectors on the drive. The operating system keeps track of where that file is stored on the drive. If, however, the file is edited and a new paragraph is inserted in the middle, the revised file may not fit neatly in its old storage location. When the file is closed after editing, the operating system may have to break it up into noncontiguous sectors, and it therefore becomes fragmented. When the user

Figure 2-12
Each user is assigned to a specific access level and is given the capabilities assigned to that level.

next retrieves that file, the OS has to go to several locations to retrieve the pieces of the file and reassemble it, which takes longer than it would had the file been contiguous.

Over time, a disk drive can become very fragmented, and file management becomes increasingly inefficient. Periodic disk defragmentation, wherein fragmented files put back together in contiguous stretches, may dramatically increase the performance of disk input-output and therefore the perceived performance (speed) of a computer.

Summary with a Note on Proprietary Versus Open-Source Software and Operating Systems

The economic issues relating to APIs and OSs are interesting and worthy of a brief discussion. Many companies, such as Adobe, make a free piece of software (i.e., the Acrobat Reader) widely available to anyone who wants it. While this seems altruistic, there are compelling economic reasons to do so. The Acrobat reader is a tool allowing the user to open and view documents conforming to the portable document format (PDF), which was defined by Adobe. To the extent that PDF has become a universally accepted standard, i.e., one which every major piece of software understands, it is successful; and the author of a document can be sure that the PDF version of that document will be accessible to anyone who wishes to look at it (using the freely available Acrobat reader).

However, software companies (i.e., manufacturer of a graphics package) wishing to provide a way to create/save a file in the proprietary or "closed" PDF format must pay Adobe a licensing fee in order to format the document in accordance with the Acrobat Reader API. The free reader generates user demand: users want software that talks PDF, and the software purveyor must pay a licensing fee to Adobe in order to meet the needs of its users.

While Windows and Apple operating systems are by far the most commonly used on personal computers, there has been a growing interest in a family of operating systems commonly known as the Linux family. While Windows operating systems are defined as closed source (like the Adobe PDF format), and therefore hidden from the consumer, Linux operating systems are open source and permit the user/consumer to see, modify, and potentially improve the original code. While most computer users are neither interested in nor capable of altering operating system code, there are any number of casual or dedicated tinkerers in the computing community who are both willing and able. The Linux community is both large and passionate about the concept of open-source code. They are constantly modifying old code and creating new code (such as new drivers) to keep the Linux operating system at the state-of-the-art.

Linux is designed to allow Unix, which is one of the progenitor operating systems, to run on personal computers. Unix was originally designed by programmers in the early 1970s as an open-source operating system that was powerful and readily adapted for different computers. Sun Microsystems used a version of Unix on its server computers, which at one time ran much of the Internet. There was a demarcation between server operating systems (Unix-based) and user operating systems (Windows and Apple). The computer savvy systems administrators who were familiar with Sun's version of Unix wanted to run something similar on their own personal computers, and a Finnish programmer named Linus Torvalds made that possible. In 1991, he posted an open source version of Unix for PCs on the web. He called it Minix. The initial version soon grew into what is now known as Linux (after Linus Torvalds) and has been under continuous modification since then. While the code for the Linux is open source, and therefore freely available, several companies (such as Redhat and Caldera) have been formed to package and distribute the Linux operating system in a convenient and easily installed package.

There are pros and cons to both the proprietary and open source approaches. Open source products, such as Linux, are usually less expensive and less fault prone than proprietary alternatives. They are less expensive by definition. They are less fault-prone if enough competent people have had a chance to examine and correct errors in the code. The bugs in Windows operating systems that have been exploited by hackers and virus programmers are fixable but went unnoticed during the development and testing periods because too few people had a chance to examine the code for flaws. Any complicated program goes through a process of maturation, during which flaws become evident and are fixed. Open source programs go through this process quickly when enough programmers identify and correct mistakes, whereas proprietary systems are closely held and the correction cycle takes longer. It is probably also safe to say that Linux is more efficient than proprietary alternatives for many of the same reasons. Unlike proprietary operating systems, Linux is designed (and continuously redesigned) to run efficiently on almost any machine. The Windows operating systems have grown dramatically in size and complexity, taking advantage of the concurrent increases in the computing power and amount of memory in successive generations of PCs.

Proprietary software has a clear advantage to the extent that software products from the same manufacturer (e.g., Microsoft or Apple) integrate seamlessly, as do Windows, Internet Explorer, and Microsoft Office. Integrated solutions (i.e., Microsoft Office) are demonstrably more desirable to users than a collection of arguably better, but unintegrated pieces (i.e., Corel WordPerfect, Harvard Graphics, Lotus 1-2-3).

Suggested Readings

Gorman M, Stubbs T. *Introduction to Operating Systems, A Survey Course*, 2nd ed. Course Technology, 2003.
Watson RA. *Introduction to Operating Systems and Networks*. New York: Prentice-Hall, 2003.

Computer Networks

What is a Network?

In its most basic form, a computer network involves a linkage between two computing devices, i.e., two computers or a computer and a printer. The number of terms used to describe various types of networks has proliferated dramatically in the past 30 years, but the fundamental principles remain unchanged. Networking implies that two computing devices have packaged the information they wish to exchange in a format both agree upon and they communicate across a shared exchange medium (such as an Ethernet connection) (Fig. 3-1).

One of the earliest "networks" was developed at Xerox's experimental laboratory in Palo Alto, California, known as the Palo Alto Research Center, or PARC. PARC's mission was the development of the "office of the future." Founded in 1970, the lab developed and patented innovative computer components including Ethernet networking, the graphical user interface later popularized by Apple, the laser printer, and spell checking. Ethernet is one of the prototypical computer networking standards, and it was developed at PARC by Bob Metcalfe. Metcalfe developed the cabling method and communication standards governing communication between an early personal computer, the Alto, and a printer. This subsequently evolved into the Ethernet standard, which has become the most popular and widely deployed networking standard in the world.

The original Ethernet standard described communications among devices on a single cable attached to all of the devices on the network (Fig. 3-2), and permitted conversations between any single device and all of the other devices (i.e., computer, printer, and so on) on that cable (Fig. 3-3).

Today's networks theoretically permit ad hoc conversations between any two users connected to the Internet at any time. Networks are now defined by security standards and firewalls rather than physical boundaries to a network. This is a miraculous concept in many regards, but as with the physiologic body, any computer can act like a cell and become the portal of entry for a virus and infect a network system.

Network Basics

Key Points

Network Terminology

- Ethernet is the progenitor network protocol.
- Local area networks (LANs) and wide area networks (WANs) are common terms used to describe the geographic extent of a network.
- There are various ways of wiring computers together such as "twisted pair," coaxial cable, and optical cable.
- Computers communicate across their connections using predefined communication *protocols* or standards.
- Computers on a network are often called nodes and they send communications in *packets*.
- Nodes (PCs) can be interconnected in a variety of ways such as in series along a cable or in a ring.
- *Repeaters* are used to amplify a signal as it travels through a network, *bridges* amplify and direct traffic through a network.

Networks can be broadly classified into two main groups, at least until very recently. LANs are typically confined within a single building, whereas

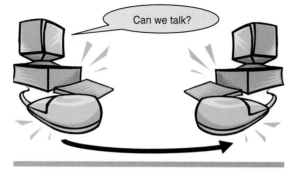

Figure 3-1
Networking requires a link between two or more computers, the mutual agreement to communicate, and a common "language."

WANs cover much larger territories and are interconnected using high-speed, high-capacity connections (Fig. 3-4). The distinctions have blurred somewhat, and, with the advent of Bluetooth technologies, in which small electronic devices can form micronetworks "on the fly," one can now think in terms of a continuum of network sizes, shapes, and capacities. Nevertheless, it is useful to consider Ethernet as prototypical networking approach for PCs (Apple uses a similar approach called Appletalk).

The original Ethernet devices networked by Metcalfe were only feet apart. Current cabling technologies, including coaxial cable, twisted pair cable and, more recently, optical cable permit devices to be tens of kilometers apart and have dramatically increased the speed of data transmission. Similarly, the first approach to packaging information for transmission between devices

was a *software* (i.e., relatively slow) approach, whereas *hardware* network interface cards (NICs) have dramatically increased the speed of network communications (Table 3-1).

The format for communication in networked devices is called the protocol, which is the set of rules that govern communication. The currency of networked communication is the packet (also called a frame or datagram), which is the basic messaging unit. It is analogous to a sentence in human communication, and has a defined structure that includes a destination and source address. There are also explicit minimum and maximum lengths to a packet. Most importantly, the packet contains a fragment of the information being passed from one device to another. Virtually all of today's networked communication uses a technology called packet switching, in which an original body of information, like this paragraph for example, is broken down into smaller elements called packets, each of which are put into an electronic envelope, "addressed," and sent from one device to another. The combination of the message and the envelope is the frame (Fig. 3-5).

The devices connected to an Ethernet are identified as nodes. Each node sees all transmissions from the other nodes. A reasonable analogy for the issues relating to networked communication is that of a meeting where there is no chairperson. When a given node wishes to "talk," the first thing it does is to listen and determine whether any other node is already talking. If there is no competition, it transmits. This leaves the possibility that two nodes could transmit at exactly the same moment, garbling the transmission of both. As with people at a meeting, Ethernet handles this eventuality by having each

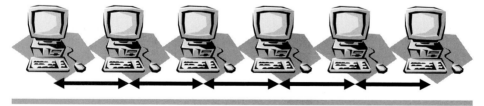

Figure 3-2
Ethernet is one of the oldest network configurations in which computers are strung along a common cable.

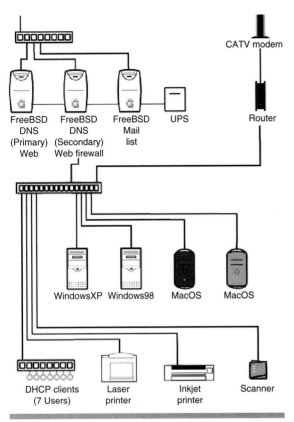

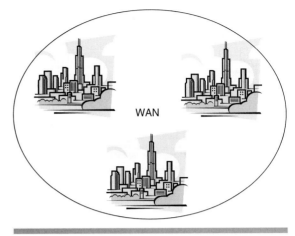

Figure 3-4
A wide area network (WAN) links widely dispersed sites often using leased, dedicated telecommunications lines.

Figure 3-3
Networks permit different devices and different operating systems to communicate using a common protocol.

node "listen" at the same time that it "talks." If a given node senses a conversational collision, it stops talking, as we would, waits a random period of time, listens again, and attempts to retransmit. It is important that there be a *random* wait, because if both nodes retransmitted after the same prescribed interval, the same collision would occur again. There are other solutions to the problem of conversational collisions, such as the one used in token ring networks, where an electronic "token" is passed sequentially among the nodes. A node wishing to

Table 3-1 Access Speeds and Characteristics of Different Network Technologies

Technology	Description	Speed	Medium	Cost/Characteristics
Dial-up modem	On-demand using plain old telephone system (POTS)	2.4–56 kilobits per second (Kbs)	Twisted pair phone lines	Cheap
ISDN	Dedicated phone line	64–128 Kbs	Twisted pair	Slighter more than POTS
Cable	Special modem and cable line needed	512 Kps to 20 Megabits per second (Mbs)	Coaxial cable	Requires existing cable access
DSL	Uses POTS	128 Kbs to 8 Mbs	Twisted pair	Asymmetric
Wireless	Wireless transmitter	30 Mbs	Airwaves	Wide area access soon to be available
Satellite	Satellite dish	6 Mbs	Airwaves	Satellite companies want to provide

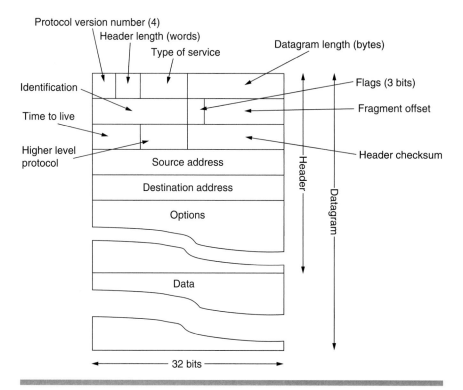

Protocol version number (4)
Header length (words)
Type of service
Datagram length (bytes)
Identification
Flags (3 bits)
Time to live
Fragment offset
Higher level protocol
Header checksum
Source address
Destination address
Options
Data
Header
Datagram
32 bits

Figure 3-5
The basic unit of communication on modern networks is the "packet," which has a header with housekeeping information and a payload or datagram with content (like a fragment of an email).

speak, takes the token out of circulation, "speaks," and then returns the token.

A number of similar analogies can be made to human communication. If there are too many nodes on a given Ethernet segment, as with too many people in a meeting, the number of conversational collisions increases significantly. If the nodes are separated by too great a distance, a statement (read transmitted packet) from one end of the room is inaudible at the other. This is due to the fact that electrical signals weaken as they travel along a cable, even an optical cable although to a much lesser degree that with electrical cable.

The limitations imposed by the constraints of the early Ethernet systems have been addressed with a number of specific innovations. Carrier-sense, multiple-access (CDMA) means that all nodes

have access to all conversations and that each node has the ability to listen (sense) and was created to enhance the efficiency of internodal communica-tion. Collision detection (CD) has already been described. The problem of communications becom-ing inaudible over long distances was alleviated by the development of repeaters, which take weakened signals from the end of one Ethernet segment, enhance them like an amplifier, and send them on to another segment. Since they act bidirectionally, repeaters can be used to increase the diameter of a given LAN. Segments can be thought of as "rooms," and while repeaters can increase the diameter of a network by connecting segments and allowing "conversations" to occur over long distances, the issue relating to the number of nodes and the poten-tial for conversation collisions remains. This last

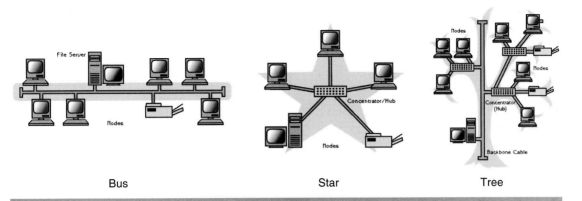

Figure 3-6
Networks can have different architectures or "topologies."

issue has been solved by replacing unintelligent repeaters with bridges.

Repeaters merely amplify the signal without addressing the problem of network congestion, whereas bridges have the capacity to filter or forward intelligently between segments. In effect, they stand at the door between two "rooms," listening to the conversations in both rooms. If a statement (packet) from an individual node in one room is intended for someone else in the same room, the bridge remains inactive. If, however, the statement is intended for someone in any another room, the bridge forward (or relays) it to the adjacent room. People (nodes) can therefore speak concurrently (without collision) as long as they are in separate rooms (on separate network segments), but bridges can route conversations among rooms. The overall effect is to permit both larger networks (more nodes on a network) and more efficient use of the network (Figs. 3-6 and 3-7).

One issue that deserves brief mention is the concept of the topology, or architecture, of a network. The earliest Ethernets had a length of cable connecting a series of nodes, which represented a single segment. Bridges were used to connect segments. More efficient communication occurred with the advent of hubs, which acted like bridges except that they were attached directly to each node in a star topology: a segment was all of the

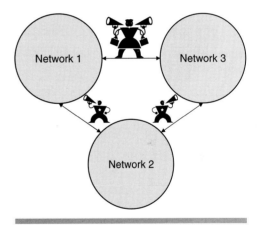

Figure 3-7
Repeaters act to amplify a signal and relay information between networks.

nodes attached to the central hub. In this arrangement, transmissions from each node were heard by and competed for "air time" with all of the other nodes on the star. Switches, while more expensive, are today's equivalent of hubs.

Most state-of-the-art Ethernet implementations today use fully "switched" Ethernet, wherein each segment consists of only a single node; every node is wired into a switch; and each switch connects to a high-speed backbone. In effect this gives every node access to a high-speed data highway, right out of the driveway as it were, as opposed to forcing it to negotiate a series of smaller capacity streets with stop signs and traffic lights on the way to the highway. In addition, whereas it was once "half-duplex," where a node could transmit or it could listen but not do both simultaneously, modern Ethernet is "full duplex." Full duplex transmission occurs when a node can listen and talk at the same time. The advent of fully switched, full duplex networks has eliminated collisions in networks so equipped, permitting each node to have reliable, consistent bandwidth.

Networking Architecture

Key Points

Evolution of Networks

- The ARPAnet was the first major network, and it was used for scientific communications.
- Ethernets were designed for intraoffice communication.
- The Internet evolved as the two distinct networks merged into one another.
- Peer-to-peer communications indicates communications between two equal computers.
- Client computers accept direction from server computers, although any one computer may take on either role in different circumstances.
- Computers communicate through virtual *ports*, which are designed for communications using specific communication protocols (like the http protocol used for web pages).

The term "network" is used to describe a group of computers connected together for communications, and the permutations of potential connection schemes have proliferated wildly. First there was ARPAnet, which was designed at the end of the 1960s—four mainframes connected together across the country for scientific purposes. It was a large WAN created by the Defense Advanced Research Project Agency (DARPA), and served as a test-bed for new networking technologies. The first two nodes that formed the ARPAnet were UCLA and the Stanford Research Institute, followed shortly thereafter by the University of Utah.

Then there was the Ethernet, which was designed for local office management. The two systems were designed for radically different purposes, and the hardware and software used to implement the two types of networks were commensurately different.

In the succeeding decades, ARPANet gave way to the Internet; and, as PCs became widely deployed in offices, small networks were developed to share access to expensive or scarce resources. In time, the two types of networks grew into one another (Fig. 3-8).

LANs were initially developed in order to enhance access to devices such as printers, disk drives, as well as to permit file sharing. Novell, IBM, Apple, Microsoft, and Unix all had products with varying degrees of usability, configurability, security, and efficiency. Novell became the dominant vendor, but later Window's operating systems have more robust networking capabilities.

There are two generic approaches to LAN management. The first is peer-to-peer (P2P), in which computers on the network communicate directly among themselves, alternating direction and accepting direction as to the management of resources, and sharing their own files and devices. This is analogous to communication between marital partners. P2P is attractive because it is simple to set up, efficient and inexpensive in small networks, and doesn't require the services of an IT administrator.

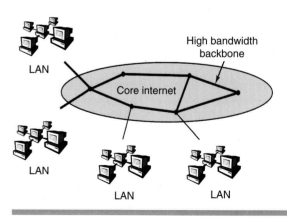

Figure 3-8
Interdigitation of the Internet backbone and LANs.

The second approach uses a network operating system which handles several core services: file sharing, printer sharing, application sharing, access control, user and resource accounting, and backup/restoring of attached devices. This is the so-called client-server approach, and more analogous to the parent-child relationship. Server-based network operating systems have an advantage over P2P because of increased security, centralization of resources, high performance, and easy maintenance. They suffer by comparison in that they are more expensive, require more expertise to maintain, and they have a central point of failure (Fig. 3-9).

The concept of clients and servers, while widely used, deserves amplification. A server requires more powerful hardware because of the communications demands placed on it. One server services requests from many clients, which may or may not be known to it. An obvious example of a client-server relationship is that of a user's browser client and the web server with which it communicates. Clients and servers communicate with one another by an agreed upon protocol, Hyper Text Transfer Protocol (HTTP) in the case of web communications. Other examples of client-server relationships are those between an email client, such as Netscape Mail, Microsoft Outlook, Eudora or Pine, and the mail server with which it interacts.

As with all client-server relationships, the same information sent from a server to different mail clients may result in very different looking outcomes. That is to say that Outlook and Eudora handle the display and management of mail differently given the exact same information from the mail server.

A server on a network may provide several services concurrently or be dedicated to one service (i.e., a web server or a mail server). A multifunctional server needs to have ways to split its communication streams so that communications intended for its web function go to the program that handles web services, while mail communications go to that function. The way this is handled universally is through the use of "ports." Ports are analogous to the jacks that switchboard operators used—an individual jack is associated with a specific function. Port 80, for example is the port used for the HTTP protocol, and port 25 is the mail port. These are some of the so-called "well-known ports" described in networking standards. There are additional ports that can be configured for specific uses on a given machine, much like there are certain radio frequencies used for weather or police communications and other frequencies that can be used on an ad hoc basis.

LANs and WANs, Intranets and Extranets

Key Points

- LANs have a common network, geographic location, and owner.
- WANs have a common network and owner, but are spread over a large geographic area and use leased communication lines.
- LANs and WANs have largely given way to intranets and extranets.
- Intranets use a combination of communication technologies, are not geographically limited but have a common "owner."
- Extranets use a combination of communication technologies, are not geographically limited, and are used to connect parties with common (i.e., business) interests.

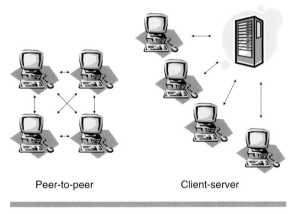

Peer-to-peer   Client-server

Figure 3-9
All computers are equal on a peer-to-peer network, whereas there are servers "talk down to" clients in a client-server network.

Table 3-2   Comparison of network types

	LAN	WAN	Intranet	Extranet
Bandwidth	High	Low	High	Low
Scope	Building/campus	City	Building/campus	City/global
Protocols	Diverse	Diverse	Internet	Internet
Security	Very high	High	Moderate	Low

The backbone of the Internet and LANs began to interdigitate in the late 1980s and early 1990s when the concept of a subnet was developed. The backbone Internet was built around five supercomputer centers funded by the National Science Foundation, while LANs were simultaneously proliferating in office settings. A set of addressing standards were developed in 1985 that married the concept of a core network (the ARPAnet) and subnetworks (Ethernets) so that they could communicate back and forth using a common language.

Network terminology has become confusing as the Internet has grown. LANs have already been described, but can be characterized as a group of computing devices connected by a common communication web (cable, switches), in a limited geographic area, using high bandwidth, sharing resources, and owned by a single entity. The shared resources include files, application software, printers, modems, fax machines, and computing power.

In contrast, a WAN is spread over a much larger geographic area, has a much larger number of devices, uses more sophisticated routing equipment and, oftentimes, leased high-speed communication links. Like a LAN, a WAN is owned by a single entity that uses the network for optimal investment in technology, to provide a single link for entity-related communication and for security.

Unlike the LAN and WAN, an intranet is defined as a network of affiliated client devices, typically operating behind a firewall and using standard internet communication protocols such as HTTP. Intranets do not have an inherent provision for sharing resources, although they are designed to share information, and there is no requirement for hardware connection.

Extranets are business-to-business intranets that are created for limited, controlled access between a company's intranet and designated, authenticated users from remote locations (Table 3-2).

Recently, new communication paradigms such as the virtual private network (or VPN) have essentially eliminated the need for LANs and WANs.

Virtual Private Networks

Key Points

- Virtual private networks eliminate the need for distinct LANs and WANs.

- VPNs encrypt communications traveling across a public network so that a secure communication link can be established between two computers or networks.

- VPNs have cut the costs of communications between traveling employees and the home office and for companies wishing to do business across the web.

- VPNs can also be used to secure communications traveling *within* a private network.

- A VPN can be used to create a one-time private link between a user and the home office or a more durable private connection between two linked entities across the Internet.

A VPN is a private network connected via, and therefore residing within, a public network infrastructure (typically the Internet). VPNs allow users to communicate via the Internet as if they were within a LAN, WAN, or an intranet. Remote users "tunnel" through the public system using encrypted, authenticated communications and appear as if they are functioning from within the remote system.

VPNs evolved as a solution to several distinct problems: an individual's need for remote access to a home system (i.e., the traveling salesman's need to remain in contact with corporate offices), the expense of dedicated high-speed connection links used in WANs and the need for security within the confines of a LAN (to permit the movement of sensitive information across the LAN).

Prior to the development of VPNs, individuals wishing to communicate with a home corporate office would need to dial in to a remote bank of modems, oftentimes paying high long-distance telephone charges in the process. VPNs allow a user to dial in to a local telephone number leased by an internet service provider (ISP) and communicate securely with the remote home office without incurring long-distance charges.

WANs were an effective way of interconnecting offices of companies with sites in multiple geographic locations, but the expense of ensuring reliable, high-speed communications among sites was often prohibitive. In addition, when a WAN was used for business interactions between two corporations, it was often unclear how to divvy up the expense. VPNs provide an attractive solution to this problem.

Finally, all machines on a LAN are interconnected by hardware and it is technically trivial for one machine to eavesdrop on traffic intended for another. Email and other sensitive information can readily be protected as it travels within the confines of a LAN by the use of the VPN paradigm within a LAN.

A well-designed VPN is secure, reliable, scales up well with the addition of new machines, and is easy to administer. VPNs come in two major varieties. The first is the VPN connection that a mobile employee uses to connect to a corporate computer environment from a remote location, such as the home or road. This function is typically outsourced today using the following model. A third party company, often called an enterprise service provider, provides phone access using either a toll free number or a bank of local (and therefore low access cost) numbers distributed geographically. The user dials into the telephone number via

modem, giving him access to the enterprise service provider's network access server, which, in turn, creates a link to the corporate VPN server. The user's VPN client software provides information authenticating the user's identity to the home corporation, and encrypts information that will be routed via the third party company. This ensures that the third party company acts only as an information carrier and is unable to "see" or alter information passing through its hands (Fig. 3-10).

Another kind of VPN is a site-to-site VPN used for fixed, secure connections among remote locations. This type of VPN is used to replace a WAN, and connects two or more remote LANs as an intranet. Alternatively, this kind of VPN connection can be used to create an extranet, in which two business partners (supplier, customer, and so on) interact via a secure, fixed (as opposed to dial-up) VPN connection (Fig. 3-11).

Some of the components used in VPNs include desktop VPN client software, dedicated VPN hardware (at the corporate end), and the network access server (maintained by the third party service provider). VPNs make use of several security features, including firewalls, encryption, authentication, access control (authorization) and accounting, but the major function of a VPN is to package information in such a way that it can be securely shipped across an insecure medium, i.e., the Internet.

Computer communications passed between two points on a VPN undergo several transformations. In the absence of a VPN connection, the original information would have passed unaltered over a network as, for example, a stream of unencoded message fragments that are reassembled at the destination computer. That same data stream is "encapsulated" for transmission across a VPN using the following series of steps. An initial message fragment, now called the passenger message, is wrapped in an encryption/encapsulating protocol or envelope (by the client VPN software on the source machine). This new, larger packet is wrapped, in turn, in a carrier packet or envelope (again on the source machine), which is the format in which it crosses the Internet to the destination machine.

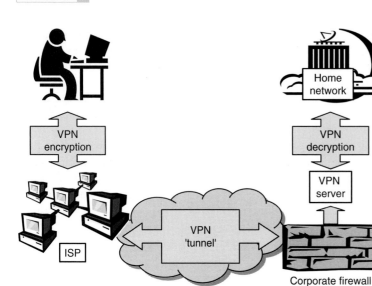

Figure 3-10
A VPN user sends encrypted communications through an ISP, across the
Internet to the corporate firewall which passes it through to the VPN
server for decryption.

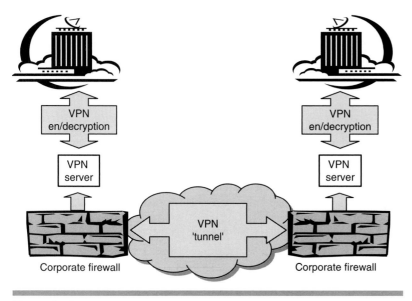

Figure 3-11
A corporate VPN allows geographically separated sites to communicate
securely as if in a single LAN.

This makes somewhat more sense when you understand what happens at the destination computer. The carrier packet was used to route the message to the destination VPN computer, which opens and discards the carrier envelope, decodes the encrypted message within, and retrieves the original message packet. The destination VPN computer can then take all of the message fragments from the original stream and reassemble them to recreate the information that went into the VPN tunnel at the source end.

Summary

Computer communication remarkably increases the ease of interaction among communities and businesses and permits the development of ad hoc secure links between businesses and clients. New communication technologies, however, bring new dangers. Much as air travel has remarkably increased potential threat of a flu pandemic, our increasing reliance on the Internet raises our vulnerability to harm originating from the network.

Communication paradigms and the definitions of boundaries around portions of the Internet are a constantly changing field. New Internet threats such as viruses and malware (described in Chap. 7) as well as increased threats to personal privacy have made the need for good "walls" and "doors" quite clear. It is no accident that the term firewall, now used in computing, derives from a building construction standard.

Suggested Readings

Hallberg B. *Networking: A Beginner's Guide*, 3rd ed. McGraw-Hill: Berkeley, Osborne, 2002.

Lowe D. *Networking for Dummies*, 6th ed. For Dummies, 2002.

McMahon R. *Introduction to Networking*. McGraw-Hill: Berkeley, Osborne, 2003.

4

Wireless Networking

Introduction

Key Points

- Existing wireless technologies include infrared, WiFi, and Bluetooth as well as the protocols used for cell phone communications.

- New technologies are developing that will permit wireless coverage over wide areas and increase the transmission speed of data.

Wireless networking is rapidly coming of age, and wireless network access is built into new portable computers as well as handheld devices including PDAs. Wireless access points are becoming available in public places such as neighborhoods and plans are underway to create wireless networks encompassing entire cities, such as one envisioned for Philadelphia.

Wireless networking technologies include infrared (which is the same technology used in TV remote controls), the WiFi family of protocols, such as 802.11b and 802.11g, and Bluetooth (Fig. 4-1). The 3G specification has been developed for cellular devices, and provides for enhanced data transfer speeds in email, instant messaging, and web browsing. It is called 3G to indicate that is the third generation of cellular communication, following the first generation analog and second generation digital. The 802 family of protocols has also been extended to provide for wide area coverage by the development of the 802.16 standard (Fig. 4-1).

Wireless networking is particularly suited to the medical environment, where providers are highly mobile and dependent on a rich stream of data generated continuously during daily activities. There are huge inefficiencies built into current approaches to patient care. A physician, nurse, or ancillary provider can spend a significant amount of time moving among patients, when access to patient data is unavailable, and then use a separate chunk of time in data acquisition and transcription. Wireless solutions have been developed for PDAs and other handhelds (described in Chap. 17) that continuously download laboratory, pharmacy, and radiographic data, eliminating the need for time specifically dedicated to data acquisition.

Wireless interfaces between devices and central servers are also becoming available. Bedside infusion pumps can store and/or forward information pertaining to alarms and rates using wireless interfaces. Many of the medical devices used at patients' bedsides, such as ultrasound, EEG, and ECG can now be equipped with wireless cards permitting them to communicate with central analysis and storage units (Fig. 4-2).

Radio frequency ID (RFID) tags are just beginning to be deployed in some hospitals and used to track patients, drugs, devices, inventory, and personnel. Implantable radio frequency identification chips have just been approved by the FDA as a way for patients to carry medical information with them at all times. A hospital or physician can interrogate the chip, given the appropriate equipment, and acquire information about allergies and prior medical encounters from patients who might otherwise be unable to provide the information due to a communication barrier.

Each of the technologies uses different wavelengths, has different bandwidths, and requires different equipment. There are specific niches for each as well and it is clear that these technologies will coexist in the hospital of the future.

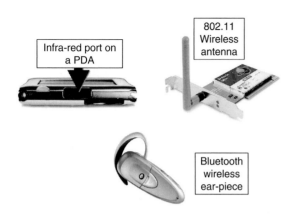

Figure 4-1
Wireless technologies include infrared, the 802.11 (WiFi) family, and Bluetooth networking.

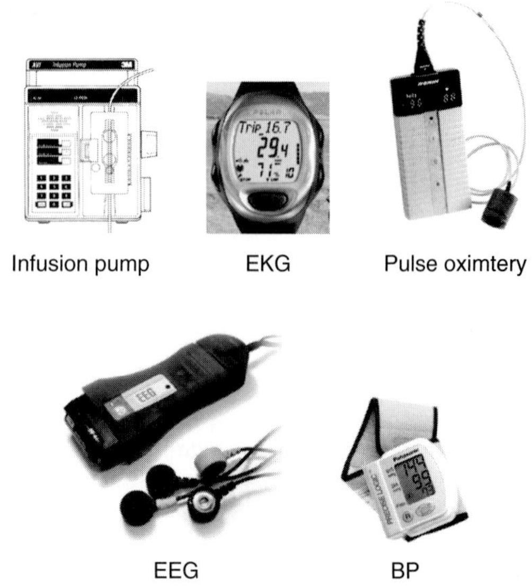

Infrared

Key points

- Infrared wireless is built into older PCs and many personal digital assistants.
- Infrared communications require an unobstructed "line-of-sight" between transmitter and receiver.
- Infrared transmissions can be interfered with by ambient fluorescent light.

Infrared, optical wireless links have been around for a while, and they are built into many devices, including most PDAs. Infrared transmitters and receivers work in the nonvisible (to humans) spectrum of light. Compared to optical communications, radiofrequency (RF) approaches (such as Bluetooth and 802.xx) suffer in that there is a potential for competition with other devices (such as telephones) among RF devices, which is not the case with optical communications. Infrared communications are limited to the confines of a line-of-sight radius, which can be advantageous from a security standpoint. It is also very convenient to point infrared-enabled devices at one another to allow them to create an ad hoc network for purposes of data transmission, such as the transaction that occurs when someone "beams" information from one PDA to another (Fig. 4-3).

Figure 4-2
Many wireless devices are now wireless enabled.

Infrared communications can have high transmission rates assuming that there is not interference from ambient light sources, such as sunlight or incandescent lamps. They may be particularly suited to certain medical environments where confidential data must be passed between devices. Some PDA-based medical applications use infrared-based synchronization to exchange patient information.

Bluetooth

Key points

- Bluetooth refers to a standardized approach for communication between or among devices including its frequency and packet structure.
- Bluetooth is designed for short range communications in an electrically noisy environment.
- Bluetooth uses an approach called frequency hopping that permits it to avoid interference from other wireless devices operating in the same range.

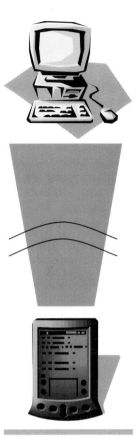

Figure 4-3
Infrared communications
require line-of-sight
visibility.

Bluetooth is a wireless communication protocol that uses a wavelength (2.45 GHz) reserved by international consensus for Industrial, Scientific, and Medical communications (the ISM frequency band). This wavelength is shared by many household devices such as baby monitors, garage door openers, and cordless telephones. While the potential for competition among these devices in many environments would seem to minimize the usefulness of a competing standard, clever technology allows Bluetooth to coexist comfortably with these devices. There are several other design features that make Bluetooth particularly attractive: it requires very little power, it is inexpensive, and

Bluetooth-enabled devices automatically sense each other and set up communications.

Bluetooth signals are very low power, 1 mW, as compared to cell phones which can transmit 3 mW signals. The signal's low power shortens the distance over which Bluetooth devices can communicate to about 10 m, although, unlike infrared, intervening walls do not block transmissions. Bluetooth-enabled devices "play well together"—many devices can communicate simultaneously in the same physical space without interfering with one another. This is possible because Bluetooth uses a technology known as frequency hopping, which was initially developed to prevent jamming of radio-controlled torpedoes during World War II (by the actress Hedy Lamarr) (Fig 4-4).

Frequency hopping involves extremely rapid, synchronized changes in frequency (within a designated frequency range, such as the ISM band) by a transmitting and receiving device. The Bluetooth protocol involves frequency shifts 1600 times every *second* in a sequence agreed upon by two (or more) Bluetooth-enabled devices that have established a network. This is kind of like a fly avoiding the rain drops. The rapid frequency shifts minimize the possibility of interference from a phone

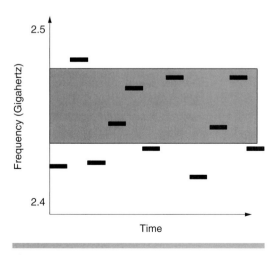

Figure 4-4
Bluetooth uses frequency hopping, with rapid
jumps within a frequency range, to avoid
interference from competing devices.

or baby monitor or another Bluetooth network operating in the same area.

Bluetooth devices establish miniature, ad hoc networks automatically using a sequence of maneuvers defined by the protocol. When a device, such as a hypothetical Bluetooth-enabled medical device, is turned on, it sends out an inquiry asking if any other devices are in the region having an address in a certain range (the one it cares to talk to). Devices fitting that description respond and create a tiny network, called a piconet. Once the piconet is developed, the devices on the piconet "frequency hop" in synchrony. In this way, several Bluetooth piconets can coexist in the same environment and not interfere with one another (since the likelihood that any two networks will be on the same frequency at the same time is very low). Bluetooth communications can proceed in one direction at a time as with a walkie-talkie (half duplex) or both directions simultaneously as with a telephone (full duplex) (Fig. 4-5).

Bluetooth applications are well suited to the medical environment. For example, it is easy to imagine a health care provider approaching a medical device carrying a (Bluetooth enabled) tablet PC

which senses the proximity of the device, establishes a piconet, and exchanges patient data and orders with the device.

Bluetooth is named after a legendary Danish king from the 900s who was able to unite portions of Denmark and Norway into a single kingdom. The Bluetooth standard was developed by a special interest group (SIG) formed by five companies (Ericsson, Nokia, IBM, Toshiba, and Intel) in 1996. Their intent was to create a communications standard that could unite the worlds of computing and telephony.

802.xx

Key points

- The 802.xx family of protocols (Table 4-1), like Bluetooth, are a series standards addressing both the frequency and structure of communications among wireless devices.
- 802.11b is known as the WiFi standard, and is quickly being supplanted by 802.11g on new laptops and other wireless-enabled devices.
- While 802.11b and g are relatively limited in their communication range, city-wide networks will soon be available using an 802.xx variant.

The 802.xx family of frequencies is a family of standards developed by the Institute of Electrical and Electronics Engineers (IEEE), which is a global society that sets standards for a variety of applications in the information technology realm. Several of the 802.11 family of standards are interchangeably referred to as

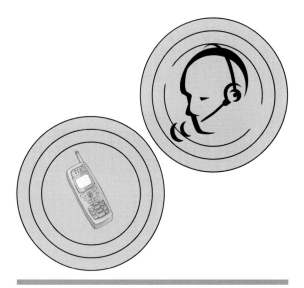

Figure 4-5
Bluetooth-enabled devices can automatically recognize the presence of other such devices and form ad hoc networks.

Table 4-1 802.xx Family of Protocols

Specification	Description
802.11	Base standard
802.11a	5.75 GHz, 54 Mbps
802.11b	2.4 GHz, 11 Mbps, traditional WiFi standard
802.11g	2.4 GHz, 54 Mbps, emerging WiFi standard
802.11i	Has security enhancements for previous stds.
802.11k	Will be used for long range (city-wide) WiLAN
802.11n	Future, very fast standard

as WiFi, but they differ in several ways, including the radio frequency that is used, transmission speed, and range.

802.11b and 802.11g

The IEEE standard for 802.11b standard is the one most commonly referred to as WiFi and built into many portable computers today. It provides 1.2 megabit per second communications, uses the 2.4 GHz range, which is the same one used by many cordless phones, and is capable of frequency hopping like Bluetooth. It was the first of the 802.11 family to come into widespread use. Paradoxically, the 802.11a standard followed 802.11b, and is significantly faster, providing for up to 54 megabits per second. 802.11a operates in the 5 GHz range (and therefore isn't interfered with by many common household devices) has not been widely deployed and is likely to remain of historical interest in that the 802.11g standard has the advantages of both 802.11b and 802.11a. 802.11g uses the 2.4 GHZ range but communicates at 54 megabits per second. 802.11g devices are also backward compatible and can therefore communicate with older 802.11b devices.

802.11e and 802.11i

802.11e and 802.11i are evolving standards designed to support the transmission of voice, video, and audio information as well as strong encryption methods. They will be used in audio and video on demand, voice over IP (VoIP) (Internet telephone), and high-speed Internet access. 802.15 is analogous to and compatible with Bluetooth communications.

802.16

802.16 is the next interesting standard that will become important to consumers. It is designed for metropolitan networks. Unlike the 802.11 family which operates over a range of 250–100 yards, the 802.16 specification refers to a family of standards designed for a range of 30 miles at 70 megabits per second. These standards are generically referred to

as metropolitan area networks (MANs). A coalition of companies in the industry including Intel and Nokia banded together in 2001 to form the WiMAX advocacy group. While transmitters and receivers conforming to this standard are not yet widely available, they will begin to become so in the next couple of years.

Related Technologies

Key Points

- RFID tags can be wirelessly interrogated or can actively signal their presence.
- RFID tags can be used for identification or tracking and have many applications in medical care.
- Voice Over Internet Protocol (VOIP) permits wireless voice communications using wireless protocols like those of the 802.11 family.
- VOIP is ideally suited for intelligent communications among medical providers.

Radio Frequency ID Tags

Radio frequency identification is the generic term for technologies that use radio waves to automatically identify objects such as products, personal identification cards, or equipment. RFID chips have been approved for subcutaneous implantation in patients.

While RFID is fairly new, there are already several approaches to RFID identification available on the market. However, the most frequently used method is to store a serial number that identifies a person or object, and perhaps other information, on a microchip that is attached to an antenna (the chip and the antenna together are called an RFID transponder or an RFID tag). This process is called RFID tagging. The antenna in the RFID tag enables the chip to transmit the identification information to an RFID reader. The reader reads the radio waves reflected back from the RFID tag into information that can be digitally sent to a computer or computer network. Software is then used to make use of the data for applications such as improved inventory control, theft deterrence, and so on.

There are two different technologies that fall under the rubric of RFID. Passive RFID either reflects energy from a reading device or it transiently absorbs the energy and then generates its own response. The energy source driving interactions with passive RFID devices is external to the device, i.e., powered by the reader, and the tag lays dormant between interactions. Active RFID devices use an internal power source to continuously power the tag, and the device can generate high-powered signals to a receiver/reader. These differences have a big impact on communication range, how many sensors can be read concurrently, and the suitability of each approach for applications in the medical environment (Figs. 4-6 and 4-7).

The communication range of passive RFID devices depends on the need for powerful signals to reach the tag. This typically constrains the effective distance between reader and tag to 3 m or less, and in some cases centimeters. Active RFID devices can be over 100 m from their associated readers. In terms of the medical implications of these limitations, passive RFID tags are being applied to prescriptions, blood samples, and even patient's ID tags, whereas active tags are being used to track expensive pieces of equipment in the hospital.

One interesting potential application of RFID tags lies in the potential to read multiple RFID tags concurrently, as one might wish to do with a cart of groceries or a box of medications. This is difficult to do with passive tags because they interfere with one another. However, thousands

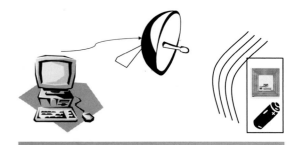

Figure 4-7
Active RFID devices "announce" themselves to antennas, but require a built-in power source.

of tags can be read simultaneously with active RFID technology.

A third difference between active and passive technologies is the amount of data that can be stored on a tag. Because of the power limitations, passive tags have limited storage capability on the order of 128 bytes, whereas active tags can store 128 thousand bytes, and can therefore be used to log events and thereby create audit trails.

Voice over IP

Voice over IP is a rapidly evolving network-based technology, in which conversations are treated as Internet data streams, which is to say that a communication link is set up between two (or more) parties over a network, and the conversation is routed back and forth in a bidirectional stream of data packets (Fig. 4-8).

Traditional phone communications involve the use of circuits, in which a caller connects to another party over a circuit that is created for the purpose of that call, maintained during the call, and then disassembled at the conclusion of the call. Using switches at telephone exchanges, the two parties to a call are effectively connected to one another over a continuous length of telephone cable for the duration of that call. In actuality, that paradigm is no longer valid, as the phone companies route a significant percentage of current phone traffic over some portion of the Internet backbone.

The original copper-wire-based conversations were analog, and therefore inherently inefficient

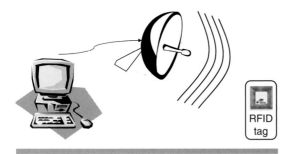

Figure 4-6
Passive RFID tags will answer when "interrogated" by a powered antenna.

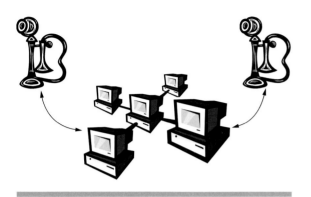

Figure 4-8
Regular phone communications can be sent across a network, which is known as voice over IP.

for several reasons. The first is the fact that the links established for the conversation were bidirectional but only half of the link's capability is used at any given time, since only one person speaks at a time. There is also a good deal of silence in most conversations, which can efficiently be eliminated or compressed for transmission. In order to realize these efficiencies, conversations must be digitized and assembled into packets and compressed.

Consider a 10-min circuit switched phone call, which would require 128 kilobit per second transmission rates to duplicate the fidelity of an analog line and obviously occupy the circuit for 10 min. Using voice digitized and packeted for transmission over IP, the same phone call would require only 3.5 min at a rate of 64 kilobits per second. In other words at least four VoIP conversations could be transmitted in the same "space" that a standard, analog, circuit-based conversation would need. Substantial additional efficiencies can be achieved by compressing the conversations [see challenge handshake authentication protocol (CHAP)].

VoIP conversations can be carried in any number of ways. There are devices by which a standard phone can be attached to a computer (wherein the analog phone signal is digitized before it is handled by the computer). There are also IP phones which are specially designed for VoIP communications. Finally, people on two different computers can talk to one another over

VoIP links using microphones. For the purposes of this chapter on *wireless* communications, it is important to consider a new, rapidly emerging application of VoIP: wireless VoIP. This technology uses phones or badges to communicate to the Internet using one of the WiFi protocols and from there to a phone. Voice recognition enhances the usability of the technology, permitting a user to speak the name of the person they are trying to reach (who may be on a regular of VoIP telephony device) to make the connection.

VoIP over wireless has been deployed in some hospitals for communication among health care workers and demonstrated significant efficiency benefits. For example, there can be substantial savings in the amount of time devoted to intrastaff communication on nursing units at a hospital equipped with a VoIP badge system. Communications are potentially faster, more direct, and overhead paging may be decreased significantly. It is easy to imagine that freeing staff from the burden of answering deskbound phones or finding another staff member on a hospital unit could result in substantial time-savings (Fig. 4-9).

Summary

Wireless networking and related technologies are rapidly evolving forefronts of computing. Whereas most network-based computing today is restricted to locations where one can plug into a network (WiFi hotspots are the obvious exception), wireless access will be widely available in the very near

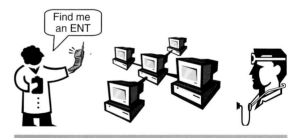

Figure 4-9
Smart communicators can be used "find" individuals or groups by name or label and establish a voice link.

future. Most medical applications of computing are currently limited by the need for wired attachments, although hospitals are rapidly developing wireless coverage.

The previous chapter described the way in which the network backbone gradually inter-meshed with local area networks and the resulting evolution of the remarkable thing called the Internet. As that network becomes freed from the requirement for wired attachments, and as wireless bandwidth increases, new and unexpected possibilities will emerge.

Suggested Readings

Lewis BD, David PT. *Wireless Networks for Dummies*. For Dummies, 2004.

Carter TW. *Wireless All-In-One Desk Reference For Dummies*. For Dummies, 2005.

5 The Internet

Introduction

Key Points

- The Internet is a rapidly growing network of networks.
- Networked connections are analogous to our roadway system.

The Internet is a global collection of interconnected computer networks, both big and small. Since its initial development in 1969, when it consisted of four host computer systems, to the present, the Internet has grown dramatically by almost any measure, although there are wildly conflicting claims as to the rate of growth. Some have stated that the Internet's size doubles every 3 months, while others suggest that it doubles only every year. The Internet was funded by the National Science Foundation (NSF) until the end of 1994 and since then its explosive growth has been a function of its inherent success.

The Internet is directly and appropriately analogous to our system of roads (or for that matter, phones, electricity, piped gas, piped water, or sewers), with small roads leading onto ever larger highways. A personal computer, for example, may link to the Internet through a cable modem, which links to a regional carrier's (such as ATT or Comcast) "point of presence" (POP). The carrier, in all likelihood, has POPs dispersed across the geographic area it serves, and each POP connects to a "network access point," or NAP. With each connection, the available bandwidth increases, much as dirt roads connect to multilane highways; and the final common pathway is the Internet backbone. The terminal or endpoint computers can make their initial connection to the Internet in a variety of ways, include a wireless connection at, for example, a wireless access point in a Starbucks, through a modem from a hotel room or from a networked computer on a LAN. Communications from all of these computers will ultimately traverse the Internet over the backbone (assuming the communications are intended for a destination that is not part of the originating network) (Fig. 5-1).

The Network

Key Points

- The organization of the core of the Internet parallels that of the telephone networks.
- Network service providers (NSPs) service the backbone of the Internet (like telephone long distance carriers).
- Internet service providers (ISP's) service the consumer and buy access to the core from NSPs (like local phone companies).
- NAPs are physical locations where backbone Internet cables and computers meet and interact.
- POPs are physical locations where the equipment of ISPs, such as the mail and web servers, are located.
- POPs need to connect to NAPs to provide their customers with access to the Internet.

The Internet can probably best be understood using a brief history of the telephone network as a background. The original telephone network was AT&T, and it existed as a monopoly, providing both local phone access and long distance connections, until its breakup in 1984. The mother company was then split into seven regional companies such as

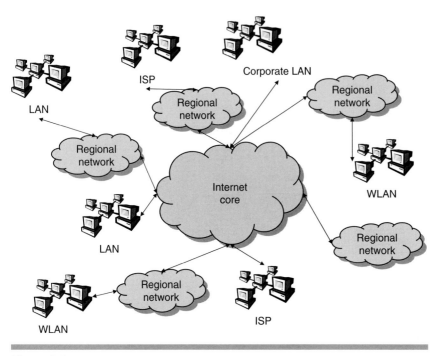

Figure 5-1
The Internet is a network of networks.

NYNEX and GTE (Fig. 5-2). What ultimately transpired was the development of *local exchange carriers* and backbone *interconnect exchange carriers*, wherein the latter serve as the long distance phone-traffic carriers for the former.

Similarly, the NSF built the NSFNET in the late 1980s as a backbone network with a hierarchical structure: regional networks connected to the backbone and local networks connected to the regional networks. When NSF privatized the network in 1994, the regional networks turned into commercial NSPs and the local networks turned into ISPs.

Like telephone-based carriers, NSPs provided backbone services or connections to the backbone and sell bandwidth to ISPs. ISPs, like telephone's local exchange carriers, sell Internet access services to subscribers, although some ISPs have become big enough to build their own networks. There is no clear-cut definition of the distinction between and NSP and an ISP, except that an ISP generally manages end-users' subscriptions and accounting services.

The original NSF backbone has been replaced by the many backboned core of the Internet, which is global, and in which there is no dominant "shareholder." Because it is in the mutual interest of all stakeholders, large and small, privately owned carriers interconnect their networks. Independent service providers such as MCI Worldcom, Sprint, Earthlink, and others have built national and global networks and sell bandwidth to smaller carriers who, in turn, resell bandwidth to even smaller entities, such as a health system. The juncture points connecting subscribers to networks and networks to one another are POPs and NAPs, respectively. These are the physical locations where cables terminate and from which routers direct computer traffic.

NAPs are Internet exchanges with open access policies serving commercial and international Internet traffic. A useful analogy is that of a large

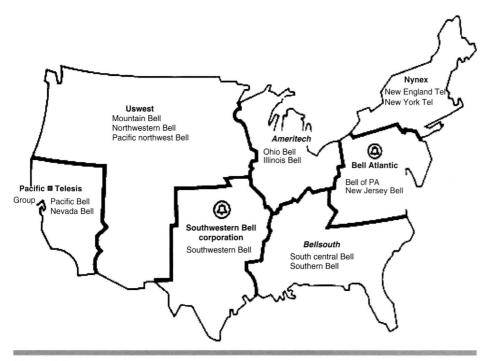

Figure 5-2
The Internet is similar to the original telephone networks in which there were regional companies that connected seamlessly to deliver communications over a wide range.

airport serving a number of independent airlines. Like an airport, in which it is economically advantageous for airlines to share common resources such as runways, baggage handling, terminal services, and so on, a NAP provides NSPs with the ability to connect to communications cables, uninterruptible power sources and switching equipment, and so on. Service providers colocate at NAPs for efficiency.

POPs are analogous to NAPs in that they are physical locations at which computers and cables come together with provisions for security, uninterruptible power, disaster protection. Unlike the equipment at an NAP, POPs are oriented to the needs of the end-user, so application-specific servers such as mail servers, web servers, and firewalls are likely to be found there. POPs may be fully owned by an individual ISP or an ISP may lease equipment and services from a POP provider (Fig. 5-3).

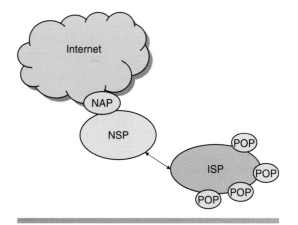

Figure 5-3
The Internet has network access points (NAPs), network service providers (NSPs), internet service providers (ISPs), and points of presence (POPs).

The efficiencies of the latter model, in which the ISP owns none of the equipment, lie in the fact that the ISP can then concentrate on selling Internet access and services (i.e., mail, web hosting) to its customers and supporting them. The ISPs leases hardware and POP access from a wholesaler in a given region. An ISP can expand into other regions merely by leasing and, in effect, act as a "virtual" ISP provider. Other specialized service providers have emerged as the Internet has grown, including application service providers (ASP), management service providers, and storage service providers. An ASP "rents" software to a subscriber and maintains the software for the subscriber. Examples of software that might be leased from an ASP include e-commerce applications, email, calendars, and so on. A *management service provider* actively monitors the customer's networks and communication links. A *storage service provider* provides disk space to subscribers with the additional benefits of security and redundancy. This service is typically used for backups or mission critical data.

Internet Packets

Key Points

- The Internet was designed to be a redundant, fault-tolerant communications system that could service local strikes to parts of the system in the event of a military attack.

- The Internet has redundant physical pathways.

- Messages such as an email are fragmented into uniform "chunks" and sent across the Internet using rules known as the transmission control protocol/internet protocol (TCP/IP) suite.

- Each fragment contains information about where it came from, where it fits in the original message, and where it needs to go, in addition to a piece of the original message.

- Missing or lost fragments are resent and the final message is the reassembled.

One of the goals of the designers of the Internet was the creation of a system that was highly tolerant of faults or breaks in the system, so as to allow the progenitor military system (DARPANet) to survive an attack. The web itself is fault tolerant in that there are multiple paths among network nodes, but the original foundation of the network's fault tolerance was the use of *packet switching* (also described in Chap. 3). Packet switching and the rules by which it is implemented ensures totally reliable, fault tolerant communications across a complicated network (Fig. 5-4).

Internet packets are typically called transmission control protocol/internet protocol (TCP/IP) packets. When a message is sent via the Internet, it is first broken into component parts of a certain size in bytes. These are the packets. Each packet carries all of the information it requires to get to its destination—the sender's (originating) address, the in-tended receiver's address, something that tells the network how many packets are in the total message, and specific the number of this particular packet (Fig. 5-5).

Packets carry the data in the form that the Internet understands: TCP/IP. Each packet contains part of the original message, which might be a piece of email, a piece of a data file or a part of a picture. A typical packet is 1000 or 1500 bytes long. After the original file is split into packets, each packet is then sent off to its destination by the best available route (as determined by a *router*). All packets in a message may take the same route or each packet may take its own route. They do not need to arrive in order: the software at the receiving end reassembles the message appropriately.

| Each packet can take separate path |
| Packets can arrive in any order |
| Missing packets are requested to be resent by receiver |
| Each packet checked for integrity on arrival |

Figure 5-4
There are several independent elements to the fault tolerance of the Internet, all of which ensure the integrity of traffic sent across it.

Header	Sender's address Receiver's address Protocol Packet #
Payload	Data
Trailer	Data to show where end of packet is Error correction

Figure 5-5
An Internet packet has three key sections including addressing information, a data section, and error correction (a check-sum).

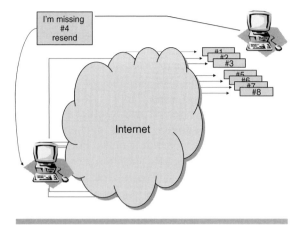

Figure 5-6
The receiving requests that a missing packet (identified by missing sequence number 4) be resent if it is not received in a certain amount of time.

The fact that messages are split and individually routed realizes several benefits. The first is network efficiency, because message fragmentation permits load balancing across various pieces of transmission equipment on a millisecond-by-millisecond basis. Second, if there is a problem with one piece of equipment in the network while a message is being transferred, packets can be routed around the problem, ensuring the delivery of the entire message. Finally, the TCP protocol ensures that each packet expected by the recipient (it knows how many total packets to expect and which ones it has received) arrives, because the recipient sends a request for retransmission of missing packets until the message is complete (Fig. 5-6).

IP is the addressing protocol used for routing packets over the Internet. The job of the IP is to permit delivery of packets across a web, where the specific route between a source and destination machine is not necessarily defined and to provide flexibility in packet size. TCP and IP work together to create a reliable, fault tolerant connection between two machines, across a network. Summarizing the way data is transmitted across the Internet, a core "message," like a piece of email, is delivered to the TCP software on a source machine by a higher level application (such as an email program). It is then fragmented by the TCP protocol into segments and reassembly information is attached to each segment. The segments are then "wrapped" into an IP envelope with destination and return addressing information. The completed packet is

then delivered into the Internet stream. The TCP software on the receiving computer reassembles the message from the packet fragments, requesting retransmission of any missing packets.

Routers

Key Points

- Internet *routers* direct the stream of Internet packets as they travel from source to destination.
- Routers "know" about how to get from one major point to another on the network, the current condition of major routes, and (in newer models) the most efficient path for a given packet.
- Routers are designed to connect portions of the network and to enhance the efficiency of the overall network by distributing network traffic and preventing "traffic jams."

On a network such as the Internet, a router is a computer that determines the next network point to which a packet should be forwarded on the way to its final destination. By definition, a router is connected to at least two networks and decides which way to send each information packet based on its current understanding of the state of the networks it is connected to. A router is located at any point where one network meets another, including each POP on the Internet. A router is often included as part of a network switch (Fig. 5-7).

A router maintains a table of available routes and their conditions, and uses this information to determine the best route for a given packet. Routers communicate with one another as to their current state of activity so that packets can be routed around over-extended nodes. For example, on Monday, the most efficient path may be from network A through network C to network B. Damage to some portion of network C, however, may favor a new path on Tuesday: network A to network D to network B. The router knows about problems on the network path, it can detour packets when appropriate. Routers talk to each other and share knowledge, such as traffic reports: "Route A is jammed right now. Take route B instead. Route C has disappeared." Intelligent routers are able to evaluate the optimal path using different metrics such as shortest path length (fewest hops from one host to another), fastest path (more hops on speedier links), or least congested path (Fig. 5-8).

Typically, a packet travels through a number of routers before arriving at its destination. One of the tools a router uses to decide where a packet should go is a configuration table, which holds information such as which connections lead to

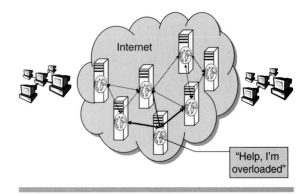

Figure 5-8
Smart routers are aware of the traffic patterns on the Internet at a given time and can route around congested areas.

particular groups of addresses, the priorities for connections to be used, and rules for handling both routine and special traffic. A configuration table can be as simple as a half-dozen lines in very small "core" routers at the edge of the Internet that have a limited number of choices as to where to send their packets. Core routers in the center of the Internet have configuration tables that grow to massive size and complexity.

A router has two separate but related jobs: The router ensures that information doesn't go where its not needed, unlike the switches in LANs which see all traffic. This is crucial for keeping large volumes of data from clogging the networks. Secondly, a router makes sure that packets make it to the best next hop on the way to their intended destination. In performing these two jobs, a router is extremely useful in dealing with two separate computer networks. It *joins* the two networks, passing information from one to the other. It also *protects* the networks from one another, preventing traffic on one from unnecessarily spilling over to the other. As the number of networks attached to one another grows, the configuration table for handling traffic among them grows, and the processing power of the router must be increased. Regardless of how many networks are attached, the basic operation and function of a router remains the same.

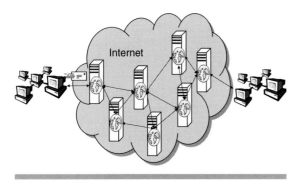

Figure 5-7
Routers have a built-in map of the Internet, which they maintain by communication among one another.

Communication Lines

Key Points

- Humans connect to the network using a variety of technologies, typically routed through an ISP's POP (see above).

- Modems are used for ad hoc connection to the network.

- "Always-on" network connections are replacing modems as the default connection to the Internet for most people.

- "Always-on" connections include integrated services digital network (ISDN), digital subscriber line (DSL), and cable modems.

- "Always-on" connections are convenient, but significantly increase the vulnerability of the subscriber to threats from the Internet.

- POPs connect to the core Internet over high capacity wire and optical cables.

The highways of network traffic are the data transmission lines and cables, and as with our system of roads, they vary in size and capacity. Many Internet connections terminate in the home and use the phone system's wires to provide the end-user with access to an Internet POP. Dial-up modems have been the access method of choice historically, but a variety of "always-on" alternatives are now available to most consumers in the United States.

Modems (modulation-demodulation devices) are designed to take the digital communications from a computer, package them for transmission over the analog lines of the telephone system for reception by another modem at the far end of the link, which recreates the original digital information. Modems have increased in speed over the last decade, and have now more or less maxed out at 56,000 bits per second (Fig. 5-9).

Two other, "always-on" alternatives are available through the phone lines. The first and older technology is ISDN. ISDN relies on a digital connection between the telephone company and the subscriber, who must be within 18,000 ft, or 3.5 miles, of the telephone company's nearest switching office

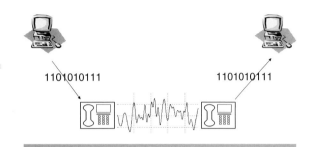

Figure 5-9
Modems take digital information from the computer, convert it to analog format for transmission across standard phone lines.

(Fig. 5-10). ISDN has a maximal speed of 128,000 bits per second (or 128 kilobits per second), and has lost market share as alternative, faster, cheaper technologies have supplanted it.

DSL is a so-called asynchronous technology, in which downstream traffic (from the Internet to the subscriber) is significantly faster than upstream traffic (Fig. 5-11). Like ISDN, DSL has a limit to the distance the subscriber can be from the central switching office and the signal degrades (becomes slower) with distance. DSL subscriptions are relatively inexpensive and easy to install. They make most sense when the subscriber is relatively close to the phone company's switching office. One of the risks of this technology is the fact that the subscriber has a so-called "fixed" IP address (See further).

Cable companies have gotten into the business of providing always-onInternet access and, as cable access has proliferated, the market share of

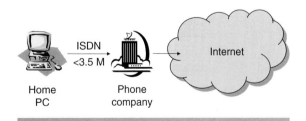

Figure 5-10
ISDN link homes within 3.5 miles of a phone company switch to the Internet.

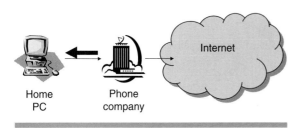

Figure 5-11
DSL links use the phone lines, and are asymmetric, sending traffic "downstream" to the user much faster than traffic from the user to the network.

cable-based Internet providers has increased. Unlike phone-based technologies, cable access is not distance limited. It is inexpensive and easy to set up and, like DSL, it is an always-on technology with a fixed IP address (Fig. 5-12). Cable subscribers also share access, and therefore access speed can deteriorate during high use periods.

The danger of computers with an always-on, fixed IP address relates to the fact that computers meeting this description are far easier to hack than devices having a dynamically assigned address. In addition, computers that are left on can be converted into drones that send out spam email or other Internet traffic under the direction of a malicious

program. This problem will be described at greater length in other chapters.

There are several other technologies that are currently or soon to be developed for Internet access including satellite connections, which are very fast and very expensive. As with DSL, these connections are asymmetric, with fast download speeds and very slow, to nonexistent upload capacity. In addition, connections may be weather limited. Wide access wireless will soon become a reality in certain environments, and as of this writing, the city of Philadelphia is planning on creating a citywide wireless access network. Because they travel through the airwaves, wireless transmissions are inherently more vulnerable than cable-based transmissions.

Most of the Internet traffic originating in a home or office ultimately passes through a commercial POP. POPs are connected to the core of the Internet by high capacity cables such as T1 (1.5 megabits per second), T3 (45 megabits per second), or optical cables. These high bandwidth cables range from megabit (T1 and T3) to gigabit per second carriage rates. To translate that into more accessible terms, it would take about 2 s to relay the entire Encyclopedia Britannica across a 2 gigabit per second optical cable.

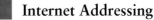 **Internet Addressing**

Key Points

- Internet addresses are used by TCP/IP packets to get from source to destination.
- Each computer on the Internet has a distinct address.
- While there are over 4 billion potential addresses using the current addressing format, addresses are running out and a new scheme is being designed which will dramatically increase the number of available addresses.
- Internet addresses have equivalents names and the two are related to the Domain Name System (DNS).
- "Root" domains include ".edu," ".com," ".gov."

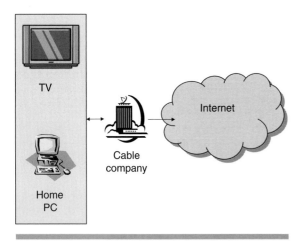

Figure 5-12
Cable "modems" send traffic over coaxial cable which is also used for television.

Internet addressing is fundamental to routing traffic from source to destination, and involves

Binary address	11011000.00011011.00111101.10001001
Dotted decimal address	216.183.103.150
Domain name	Myaddress.com

Figure 5-13
Internet address formats.

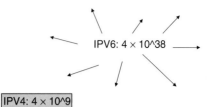

Figure 5-14
The number of possible addresses in the new IPV6 is unimaginably larger than the currently available addresses in IPV4.

the complicated interplay between the addresses we humans understand, such as "aol.com" or "yahoo.com," and the binary, bit-based, numeric format understood by machines, such as the following: 11011000. 11101111. 00100101. 01100011. That address translates to an IP address of 216.239.37.99, which is owned by "google.com" (Fig. 5-13).

Since it is obviously problematic for two machines on the Internet to have the same address. (Traffic intended for either machine would then go to both), every machine has a unique address. The number of potential address available on the Internet is a function of the binary format in the previous paragraph. The Internet address is divided into four parts separated by periods. Each part has eight positions, which can be occupied either by a 1 or a 0. The binary addresses correspond to digital addresses from 0.0.0.0 to 255.255.255.255, and allow for 4,294,967,296 potential unique addresses. While this would seem to be more than adequate for all of the potential addresses the Internet would ever need, it has become clear that this address "space" is soon to become insufficient, and new addressing modes will be required, and new generation of the IP addressing approach is under development called IPversion 6, which will replace the current version (4), which is 20 years old. The new version will have 340 trillion, trillion, trillion addresses (Fig. 5-14).

How, then do Internet messages find their way across the infinitely complicated web that it has become. When the Internet consisted of a small number of machines, users knew the raw IP addresses of the machines with which they wished to communicate, much as we might know the telephone numbers of a core group of people we call frequently. As the Internet grew, its stewards developed a way to equate text-based names with numeric IP addresses, and in 1983, the University of Wisconsin created the domain name system (DNS). The domain name server handles all requests to translate a domain name to a numeric IP address. Name servers do two things all day long: they accept requests from (1) programs to convert domain names into IP addresses and (2) other name servers to convert domain names into IP addresses (Fig. 5-15).

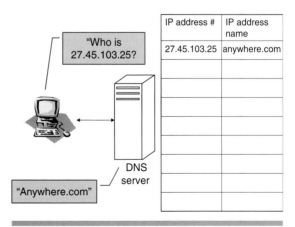

Figure 5-15
A domain name server knows how to connect address names and numbers, like a phone book.

When it receives a request, the name server does one of several things:

- It can provide an IP address because it already knows the correct address for the queried domain.

- It can contact another name server to find the IP address for the requested name. It may have to do this multiple times using alternative name servers it knows about.

- It can say, "I don't know the IP address for the domain you requested, but here's the IP address for a name server that knows more than I do."

- It can return an error message if it determines that the requested domain name is invalid or does not exist.

Domain name servers are distributed throughout the Internet, and some of them know many names, such as the "root servers" in the heart of the Internet, whereas other are familiar with a limited number of local addresses.

When a name like yahoo.com is typed into a browser's address line, its first step is to convert the domain name and host name into an IP address so that the browser can request a Web page from the machine at that IP address. To do this conversion, the browser has a conversation with a name server. A name server is also contacted when you send a piece of email to a domain address, i.e., to someone@yahoo.com. One of the first things that a new computer on the Internet will need to know is the address of a nearby domain name server (DNS).

Domains are stratified into different levels. The original seven levels will be familiar to most readers, and include .com, .edu, .org, .net, .gov, .mil, and .arpa (Fig. 5-16). Seven more root names have been added recently and they are: .aero, .biz, .coop, .info, .museum, .name, and .pro. As you can see in figure, the hierarchy in a domain name reads from left to right, which is to say that the portion of the name that is highest in the hierarchy is the rightmost portion, i.e., .com. In reading the news at yahoo, you communicate with the server residing at "news.yahoo.com." The news server resides within the yahoo domain, which, in turn, resides within the .com domain. These constructs

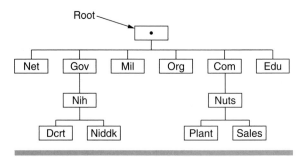

Figure 5-16
Internet extensions are hierarchical as: "*.niddk.nih.gov."

apply to the U.S. domain system, in which no final modifier is used. Domains residing elsewhere have a country specific domain indicator in the final position; while there is a "www.amazon.com," which is the American web site, the British counterpart is "www.amazon.co.uk."

Summary and Future Nets

Key Points

- Demands on the Internet are growing exponentially.
- Two "new" Internets are under development: the Next Generation Internet (NGI) (governmentally funded) and Internet-2 (academically funded).
- The new Internets are designed to dramatically increase the speed of transmission of data across them.

As the Internet has grown in complexity and the diversity of its functions, new demands have been placed on it with the advent of processes like voice over IP (VOIP), Internet radio and television. The data streams associated with these functions can be handled in several ways. A common way for "one way" streams, like radio and video, is for the radio or video server to first determine the available bandwidth between itself and the user's machine. Having done this, the server sends enough material downstream to the user that a buffer is filled. The buffer is analogous to a water tower, which is constantly filled by a pump and emptied by consumers, and the filling and consumption can occur at different rates with no perceptible drop in water pressure because the tower buffers the town from the pump and vice versa. The buffering approach is obviously unsuitable for voice over Internet phone calls: the two (or more) parties to a phone call need to be able to converse interactively. VOIP protocols take advantage of concepts like "packet prioritization," in which voice packets are given a higher routing priority than, for example, HTTP or email packets, since there is no major price to be paid for minor delays in the transmission of the latter. VOIP and other applications, such as remote surgery for example, have an inherent need for a guaranteed quality of service for connections. For example, a surgeon operating from a remote location using robotic tools must have essentially real-time feedback from his instruments to operate effectively.

Today's Internet is too slow and unreliable for applications such as remote surgery. Two efforts are underway to create the next generation of the Internet. The creators of these networks envision the use of interactive three-dimensional environments with omnidirectional sound and dazzling graphics. The research, commercial and educational possibilities are mind-numbing. One project is known as NGI, whereas the other is Internet-2.

Like the first Internet, NGI is a governmentally founded and funded effort, including the Defense Advanced Projects Agency (DARPA), the Department of Energy, the National Science Foundation, the National Aeronautics and Space Administration (NASA), and the National Institute of Standards and Technology. The NGI is already complete, although limited to a small number of locations. NGI is approximately 1000 times faster than the Internet.

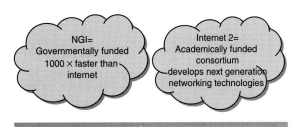

Figure 5-17
There are several next generation Internet efforts designed to identify new technologies for faster communications.

Unlike NGI, Internet-2 is university based and has 207 participating universities (as of this writing) including Stanford, the University of California at Berkeley, Harvard, Cornell, Yale, Princeton the University of Pennsylvania, and the University of Virginia. Corporate partners include AT&T, IBM, Microsoft, Cisco, and MCI. Internet-2 also receives funding from NGI, so the two are interlinked. Like NGI, Internet-2 envisions a gigabit network that will permit the transmission of massive datasets, such as the Encyclopedia Britannica, across the network in seconds (Fig. 5-17).

As routing and cabling technology advances, new applications will become possible and compel the development of succeeding generations of the Internet.

Suggested Readings

Gralla P. *How the Internet Works*, 7th ed. Indianapolis: Que Publishing, 2003.
Comer DE. *The Internet Book: Everything You Need to Know About Computer Networking and How the Internet Works*, 3rd ed. New York: Prentice-Hall, 2000.
Levine JR, Young ML, Baroudi C. *The Internet for Dummies*. For Dummies, 2003.

6

The Browser

History

Key Points

- The browser-based Internet was "invented" by Tim Berners-Lee.
- Marc Andreessen created the first widely used "browser" which eventually became Netscape.
- The Internet Explorer (IE) was a "copy-cat" Microsoft product that eventually eclipsed Netscape.

The "invention" of the Internet browser is assigned to various individuals depending on who one reads, but true credit belongs to Tim Berners-Lee at the European Organization for Nuclear Research, commonly known as CERN. Written at the end of 1990, the first browser was released in early 1991 and spread through the high-energy physics community (the people who interacted with CERN) as a communication tool for the Internet which had previously relied on a so-called "command line" interface (Fig. 6-1).

Berners-Lee's browser was written for the NeXT operating system (NeXT was a company run by Steve Jobs in the 1990s) and other browsers were subsequently written for Unix and Macintosh systems. However, it was the 1994 release of the Mosaic/Netscape browser that marked the beginning of the Internet age.

While at the National Center for Supercomputing Applications, Marc Andreessen wrote the Mosaic browser for Unix in 1993. This browser was subsequently licensed to Netscape Inc., founded by Andreessen and Silicon Graphics founder Jim Clark, which went public with beta releases of the Netscape browser in 1994. Netscape had a graphical user interface (GUI) and relied on the hypertext markup language (HTML) to communicate from a client (the user's computer) to a server (i.e., Yahoo) computer over the Internet (Fig. 6-2).

Netscape's stock soared on the day it was released and many assign the start of Internet boom to that date. Microsoft was slow to react to the release of Netscape, and Bill Gates initially viewed the Internet as a short-lived phenomenon. However, the company subsequently developed internet explorer (IE), which it released as a free component of its Windows 95 operating system (in 1995). Netscape led the innovation in browser features during a series of rapid paced releases of new browser versions during the mid-1990s. Some of its breakthrough features included frames (the "windowpanes" in current generation browsers), incorporation of Java and Javascript (industry standard browser programming tools) into the functions of the browser, and the development of the "plug-in" paradigm (by which information such as files, video, animation, and sound are handled directly through the browser rather than a separate program) (Fig. 6-3).

IE has steadily gained market share since 1995 to the point that it is now far and away the predominate browser on machines with Windows-based operating systems. Parenthetically, the pace of browser innovation has slowed dramatically during the same period. A new browser, the Mozilla Firefox browser, has recently been released and is equipped with a number of attractive new features (such as tabbed browsing) that are likely to reinvigorate browser innovation.

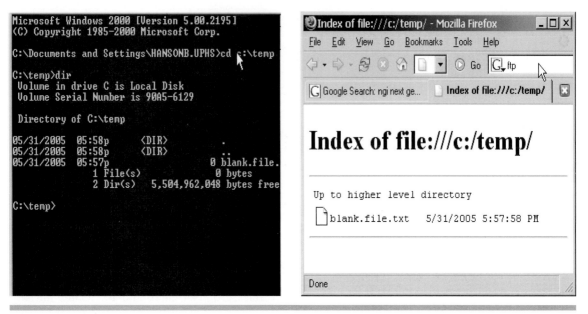

Figure 6-1
The command line (left) interface differs significantly from the windowed (right) interface to the operating system.

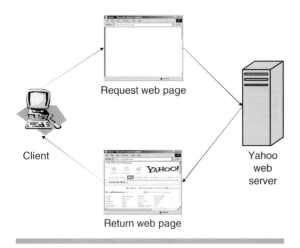

Figure 6-2
Browser communications involve a request to a server from a browser "client" on a PC—the server sends content in response.

How a Browser Works

Key Points

- The browser is a piece of software analogous to a TV screen.
- The browser displays content in the way it is told to by a language called HTML.
- The client (read your) computer communicates with a server (like Yahoo) computer during web browsing.
- There are other mark-up languages (such as those used by wireless devices) each of which is designed to direct the layout of text and pictures on a "screen."
- A web page must reside on a computer that can act as a server to be seen on a network.

There are three essential components to web browsing: the browser (which is a GUI for web communication), HTML (which is the basic language used for web communication), and the

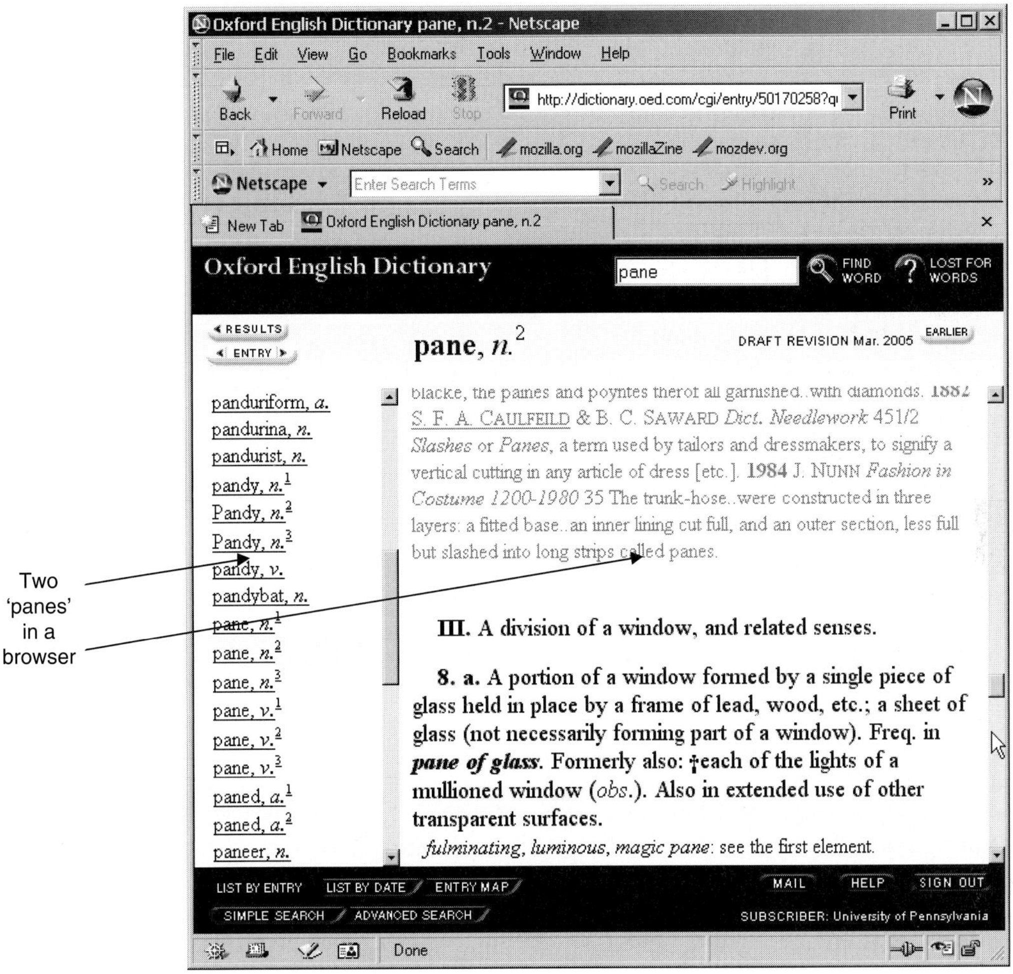

Figure 6-3
Netscape pioneered the concept of "panes" in a browser window.

client-server personal computer pair (the two parties in the "conversation").

The browser is a computer program with a GUI that has two fundamental functions: (1) it knows how to find a web server somewhere else on a network and request a copy of a file from it, and (2) it knows how to translate that file into a web page using the contents of the file, which are typically hypertext markup tags defined by the HTML. It is sort of like a TV screen—it displays content when the content it receives comes in the right format.

The term "markup" is not new, and actually relates back to word-processing, which was one of the original functions on stand-alone computers. An example of a markup might be <p>, which could indicate "start new paragraph" to a word-processing program. Any document formatted by one of today's word-processing programs has a large amount of, typically hidden, formatting information pertaining to type size, font, and paragraph management embedded in the document, without which the text would look like one long run-on paragraph.

HTML is a mark-up language specifically designed for web pages and one which has gone through a series of generations. It is a consensus recommendation from the World Wide Web consortium, and is generally adhered to by all of the browser development teams (Fig. 6-4). The current version of HTML is HTML 4.0, although there is a so-called HTML 5 which is also known as the extensible hypertext markup language (XHTML or XML). HTML was designed at CERN for the exchange of files and data, and has been creatively modified (or what the programming community would call "hacked") over the years into its current format. While HTML is serviceable, it was clearly time for a bottom-up rewrite of the *lingua franca* of the web which resulted in the recent development of XML.

Without getting into the specifics, XML is a structured set of rules used to define sets of data to be shared on the web; HTML can be thought of as one such set and has been reformulated as XHTML. As long as a web client (your phone, for example) and a web server (at your phone company) agree on the rules, they can communicate efficiently using that set.

As it turns out, HTML is not efficient for Internet communication using phone-based browsers, and another subset of XML, wireless markup language (WML or XWML), was designed for this purpose. In the near future, the majority of Internet access will be carried out on non-PC platforms such as palm computers, televisions, refrigerators, automobiles, telephones, and so on. In most cases these devices will not have the computing power of a desktop computer, and will not be able to accommodate the inefficiencies of HTML during client-server communication.

For our purposes it is reasonable to look at HTML as a general example of a markup language, and examine the way in which it is used to determine what a web page looks like. The generic formatting element is the HTML tag or programming code. The browser takes an HTML document, parses it for tags, does what the tags indicate, and displays the resulting document. The tag is distinguished from regular text by its enclosure in brackets. For example, <body> (or <BODY>) is used to indicate that what follows is "body text." Most tags come in matched pairs, where the inclusion of a forward slash in the angle brackets indicates the closing element: <BODY> indicates the start, and </BODY> the end of a section of body text.

There are some required elements in any HTML document, including <HTML> to indicate that what follows is an HTML document, <HEAD> to indicate that what follows is the page header, <TITLE> to indicate the start of the title of the page, and <BODY> to define the beginning of the body of the page. Each of these required elements has a matched closing element: </TITLE>, </HEAD>, </BODY>, and </HTML>. Note the order of the closing tags in the previous sentence: the opening and closing <html> tags surround the entire document, while the head and title sections come before the body. Tags that are out of order will result in an ill-formed or nonfunctioning web page (Fig. 6-5).

The HTML underlying any web page can be seen using a browser function which can be accessed by right clicking at some point in a web page and choosing "view source" or "view page source" (depending on the browser). The browser will then "reveal" the underlying HTML code and text that directs the appearance of that web page. It is very simple to create an html document using a text editor like the one included with the Windows operating system called Notepad. For example, to create a simple web page, you could open Notepad and type the following text into a document:

```
<html>
<head>
<title> A Simple Web Document </title>
</head>
<body>
This is Body text
</body>
</html>
```

Once created, you can save this as a file called web_page.html. If you open the file with a web browser, the resulting page will look like (Fig. 6-6).

```
<li><tt>Teletype</tt> text</li>
<li><em>Emphasized</em> text</li>
<li><strong>Strongly emphasized</strong> text</li>
</ol>
<p>This one uses lowercase alpha characters and starts at 30:</p>
<ol type="a" start="30">
<li><u>Underlined</u> text</li>
<li><strike>Strikethrough</strike> text</li>
<li><i>Italicized</i> text</li>
<li><b>Bold</b> text</li>
<li><tt>Teletype</tt> text</li>
<li><em>Emphasized</em> text</li>
<li><strong>Strongly emphasized</strong> text</li>
</ol>
<p>This list uses uppercase alpha characters and starts at 12:</p>
<ol type="A" start="12">
<li><u>Underlined</u> text</li>
<li><strike>Strikethrough</strike> text</li>
<li><i>Italicized</i> text</li>
<li><b>Bold</b> text</li>
<li><tt>Teletype</tt> text and a sublist:
   <ol type="a">
    <li>An item</li>
    <li>Another item
      <ul>
        <li>&lt;ul&gt; item a</li>
        <li>&lt;ul&gt; item b</li>
        <li>&lt;ul&gt; list item c, which contains two &lt;hr&gt;s
          and an embedded list
          <hr />
          <ol start="37">
            <li>Deeply nested item one</li>
            <li>Deeply nested item two</li>
            <li><a href="#tomjones">The excerpt from <cite>Tom
              Jones</cite></a> is a link to an earlier section of
              this document.</li>
```

Figure 6-4
This is a sample of the HTML language.

This shows the use of the key html tags. There are tags for text formatting, including color, size, font, bold, italics, and underline. Additional tags are for paragraph formatting, and management of background color. For example, by modifying the previous html file to read:

```
<html>
<head>
<title> A Simple Web Document </title>
</head>
<body>
```

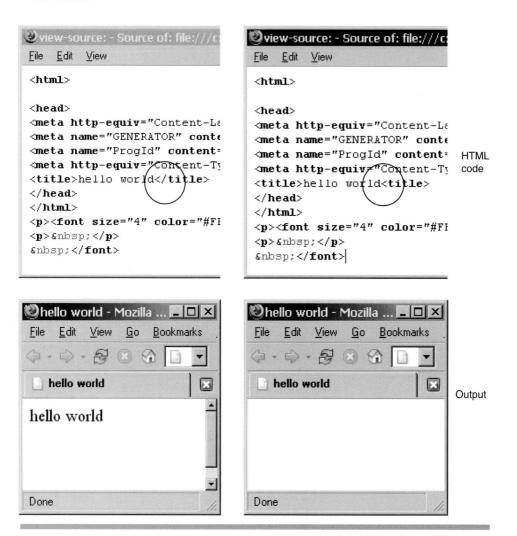

Figure 6-5
Note that the absence of a single character (/) in the html code on the right makes the web page non-functional.

```
<body bgcolor="green">
This is <font color="blue">Body </font> text
</body>
</html>
```

The resulting page will look like (Fig. 6-7).

Additional, more sophisticated, tags are designed to permit the creation of lists, links, email links, images, graphics, tables, and frames. These tags can be used to design creative and functional web pages.

Early web page designers were required to learn the html language and code their own web pages. Today, much of the complexity of web page designing has been eliminated by the evolution of user-friendly, web page design programs, or html editors, like Microsoft Frontpage or Publisher (which are bundled with Microsoft Office) and

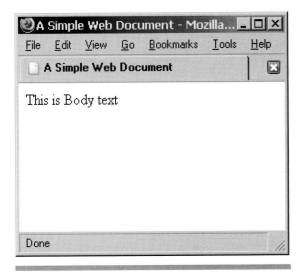

Figure 6-6
The code on the left results in the page on the right.

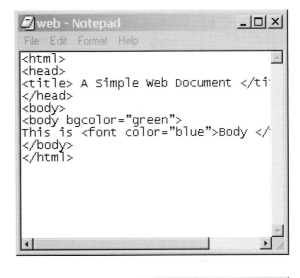

Figure 6-7
Minor modifications of the code in figure 6-6 result in more interesting and colorful web pages.

Mozilla Composer (which is a free download). These programs allow one to create web pages, and debug them interactively to evaluate the look and feel of the page on the fly.

The mere creation of a web page is not sufficient to make it a part of the Internet. You can view an html document that is stored on your own computer, but no one else can unless your computer is linked to the Internet and is also acting as a server,

therefore permitting public access to some of its file space. Many people "upload" their web pages to a web hosting service provided (often without charge) by many institutions, commercial services, and universities. Some of the "free" services require display of a commercial banner (advertising that service) on web pages they host. An alternative which permits more flexibility in the use of space,

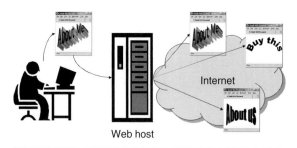

Figure 6-8
A user can create a personal web page on the Internet using a web hosting service, which is provided by many ISP's.

higher reliability, and greater speed, is to pay for web space (Fig. 6-8).

Having set up a web page, many people wish to maintain statistics on how many times the page has been accessed and from where. Services such as Show Stat, Site Meter, or Web Trends can be used to acquire site access statistics.

How a Browser Interacts with You

Key Points

- Java, Javascript, ActiveX, and common gateway interface (CGI) represent various enhancements to basic HTML permitting greater degrees of creativity and interactivity in web pages.

- Cookies are used by web servers to keep track of its interactions with a user both within a given session and between sessions.

- Popups and popunders represent relatively benign examples of actions a browser can perform without a user's request.

- More malignant unrequested behaviors have become common as vulnerabilities in Java, ActiveX, and other browser languages have been exploited by malicious programmers.

By itself, the html language is limited in that it only permits the development of static (lacking "bells and whistles") web pages, although admittedly with hot links to other pages. This degree of functionality was an enormous advance at the

inception of the Internet. However, it has been the development of our ability to interact dynamically using web pages that has permitted the boom in Internet commerce, banking, advertisement, and so on. A typical interaction involves the submission of information from a user to a web-based application. For example, when you perform an Internet search, you "submit" the search terms to the search engine. Similarly, when you engage with a commercial site (i.e., Amazon), you exchange information with that site rather than passively viewing it.

A number of different mechanisms have been developed to add interactive capabilities and functionality to web pages and a few of the most common ones are described below.

Java Programming

Java is a programming language designed for use in the Internet environment. It was introduced by Sun Microsystems in the mid-1990s, and has a number of characteristics that make it ideal for programmers to develop tools by which a user can interact with a browser and/or web page (Fig. 6-9).

```
/*
 * 1.0 version.
 */

import java.awt.*;
import java.util.*;
import java.applet.Applet;

public class AppletButton extends Applet implements R
    int frameNumber = 1;
    String windowClass;
    String buttonText;
    String windowTitle;
    int requestedWidth = 0;
    int requestedHeight = 0;
    Button button;
    Thread windowThread;
    Label label;
    boolean pleaseCreate = false;

    public void init() {
        windowClass = getParameter("WINDOWCLASS");
        if (windowClass == null) {
            windowClass = "TestWindow";
        }
```

Figure 6-9
Java code differs from HTML and can be used to design functional web elements such as buttons.

The first positive aspect is Java's similarity to a programming language widely used for application development called C++. Because Java and C++ share many similarities, it is not difficult for a programmer to learn both. Both languages, for example, are well suited for what is known as "object-oriented programming."

Object-oriented programming derives its name from its reliance on the description of objects as well as their actions and interactions with other objects. One could, for example, model the human body using the object paradigm, where each organ is characterized as a separate object. A programmer could make a simple model of the heart by describing two variables, heart rate and stroke volume, and two "methods," "change heart rate" and "change stroke volume." The heart object could then interact with other organ objects and the behavior of the human body could be described to some degree of preciseness.

A second attractive feature of Java programming is that it is very easy to implement in various environments. All of the major browsers are capable of running Java programs or small applications known as applets. All of the operating systems also run Java programs. The benefit of this universal applicability is the fact that applications written in Java will run on essentially any combination of operating system and browser. Java applets are widely used in web programming, as are closely related elements called Javabeans.

Finally, Java programs are designed to be very secure, preventing inappropriate interactions between a web-based application or the browser and the user's computer, an issue that is of growing concern as we'll see when we discuss adware and spyware (Chap. 7).

Javascript

Javascript was developed by Netscape, and was designed to provide programmers with a simple way to do things in web pages that are not provided for with the html language (Fig. 6-10). Unlike Java, Javascript programs and commands are interpreted, which means that they are broken down into instructions that the computer hardware can understand as they are encountered (rather than "compiled" prior to deployment). This makes for more programming flexibility, but means that these programs may run slower than Java programs. For example, Javascript programs might be used to cause a popup window to appear when one clicks on a hot link.

ActiveX

An ActiveX control is similar to a Java applet. Unlike Java applets, however, ActiveX controls have full access to the Windows operating system and can control resources or how your computer behaves. This gives them much more power than

```
<APPLET CODE="ripple" width=118 height=89>
<param name="image" value="day.gif">
<param name="period" value="25">
<param name="frames" value="12">
<img src="day.gif" width=118 height=89 >
</applet>

<p align="center"><font face="arial" size="-2">Free Java applets
provided by</font><br>
<font face="arial, helvetica" size="-2"><a
href="http://javascriptkit.com">JavaScript
Kit</a></font></p>
```

Figure 6-10
This javascript code can take a normal image and give it ripples.

Java applets, but with this power comes a certain risk that the applet may damage software or data on your machine. To control this risk, Microsoft developed a registration system so that browsers can identify and authenticate an ActiveX control through a trusted third party before downloading it. This assumes that the third party has correctly designated the author of the ActiveX control as trustworthy. Another difference between Java applets and ActiveX controls is that Java applets can be written to run on all operating systems, whereas ActiveX controls are currently limited to Windows environments (Fig. 6-11).

While ActiveX is a technology that permits a web page author to create impressive, interactive web content, its inherent power can potentially allow a malicious or clumsy author to do bad things to someone else's (read your) computer.

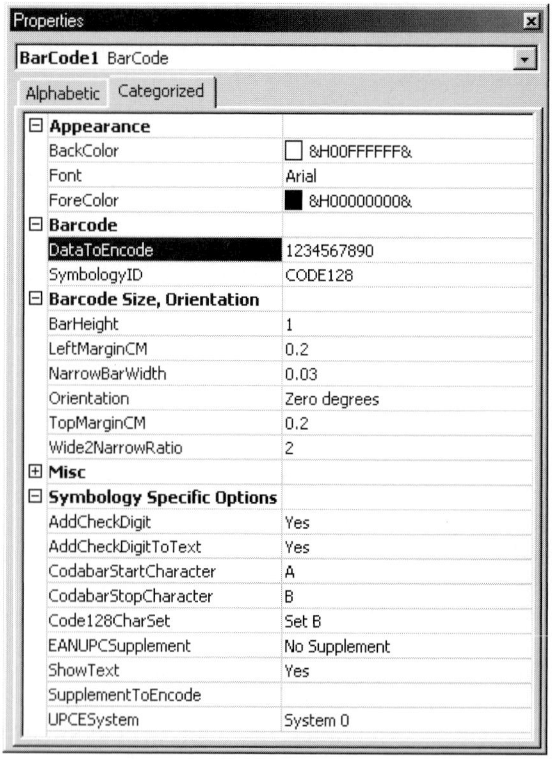

Figure 6-11
ActiveX is a Microsoft product, which can be used to add functionality to a web page.

This will be more extensively treated in the section on adware and spyware.

CGI Scripting

Like Java, Javascript, and ActiveX, the CGI is another way for a web user to interact with something other than a static web page. As indicated earlier, the typical interaction between a browser and a server is a browser request for a file (a static, html encoded web page) from the server, which retrieves the file from its disk space and sends it back to the client browser. The CGI allows the server to interact dynamically with the user. One very typical use of dynamic, CGI-based transactions occurs when you interact with a search engine (Fig. 6-12).

In a search, the end-user requests the home search page (such as the Google search page) from the search engine server, and uses it to enter search terms. The server then "dynamically" uses those search terms (by running a program) to find the requested material, repackage it, and send it back in a new web page to the user. This kind of interaction is very typical of any web transaction that uses "forms," such as searches and questionnaires.

The CGI application at the server end is a program which can be programmed in almost any programming language; and, as long is it conforms to certain requirements, the program can be quite flexible. The programs are written to take material from the form, such as the search terms entered into a search engine, and then do something, typically return a new or modified web page to the user.

Additional Plug-Ins

The "plug-in" paradigm permits a wide variety of interactions between the browser and a server, but assumes that the browser is equipped with the plug-in and the server has the appropriate server-side software. Plug-in applications are programs that can easily be installed and used as part of your browser. The early Netscape browsers allowed one to download, install, and define programs that played sound or motion video or performed other functions. These were called "helper" applications. However, these applications ran as a separate

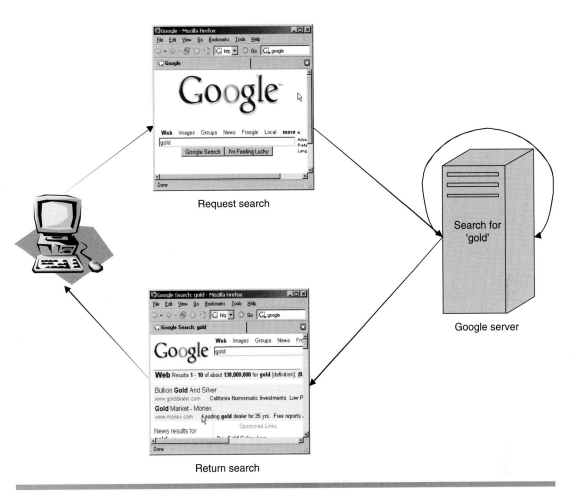

Request search

Search for 'gold'

Google server

Return search

Figure 6-12.
CGI is often used to pass form-based information back and forth between a client and a server.

application and required that a new window be opened. A plug-in is recognized automatically by the browser and its function is integrated into the main HTML file that is being displayed by the browser.

Popular plug-ins that should be familiar to most users include Adobe's Acrobat, a document presentation and navigation program that lets you view documents just as they look in the print medium, RealNetworks' streaming video player, the Windows Media Player, Quicktime (from Apple) and Macromedia's Shockwave, an interactive animation and sound player. There are now hundreds of possible plug-ins. Most users will not install a plug-in until it becomes necessary for

interaction with a web site, which will typically offer to download the plug-in to the user. Users can see the plug-ins installed in their browser as shown in (Fig. 6-13).

Cookies

Cookies are what might be called markers used by the Internet server to remember things about the users with which it interacts. Without cookies, for example, each time you refresh a web page, the server forgets who you are and what you've done during that session. Cookies are used to automate registration at a web site so, for example, you can

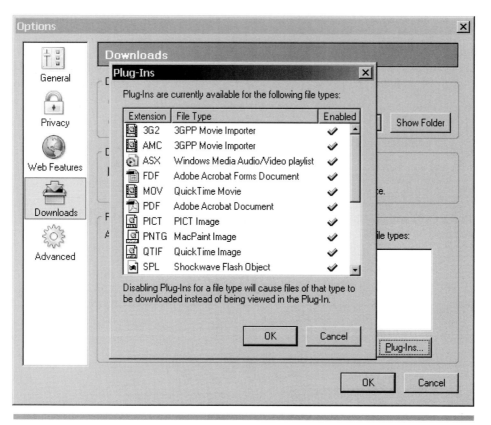

Figure 6-13
A browser can be "equipped" with plug-ins allowing it to interact with proprietary formats (like Adobe) and display the content within the browser window.

browse directly to the personalized "My Yahoo" rather than the generic Yahoo home page.

The concept of a cookie was, like many other browser innovations, introduced by Netscape. According to an article written in 1997,

> Lou Montulli, currently the protocols manager for Netscape's client product division, wrote the cookies specification for navigator 1.0, the first browser to use the technology. Montulli says there's nothing particularly amusing about the origin of the name: 'A cookie is a well-known computer science term that is used when describing an opaque piece of data held by an intermediary. The term fits the usage precisely; it's just not a well-known term outside of computer science circles.'

A good analogy for a cookie is used by David Whalen, the author of "*The Unofficial Cookie*

FAQ (Frequently Asked Questions)," which can be found at www.cookiecentral.com. He likens a cookie to a laundry ticket: "You drop something off, and get a ticket. When you return with the ticket, you get your clothes back. If you don't have the ticket, then the laundry man doesn't know which clothes are yours. In fact he won't be able to tell whether you are there to pick up clothes or a brand new customer. As such the ticket is critical to maintaining the state between you and the laundry man. HTTP is a stateless protocol. This means that each visit to a site (or even clicks within a site) is seen by the server as the first visit by the user. In essence, the server "forgets" everything after each request, unless it can somehow mark a visitor (that is, hand him a "laundry ticket") to help it remember. Cookies can accomplish this."

Another good reference source for information about cookies is the "Howstuffworks" site: www.howstuffworks.com. Marshall Brain, the author of the web site's article on cookies, characterizes some of the inaccurate information about cookies in the following paragraph:

> Cookies are programs that Web sites put on your hard disk (not). They sit on your computer gathering information about you and everything you do on the Internet (they don't), and whenever the Web site wants to it can download all of the information the cookie has collected (it can't).

While these preconceptions may be accurate for some of the newest Internet viruses, they are completely *inaccurate* as regards cookies.

Cookies are typically very simple strings (lines) of text that a Web server stores on the user's machine with the user's browser. The text lines may contain generic information, like an anonymous user ID assigned to you. Note that this ID is assigned to you on your current browser and on your current PC; which is to say that if you use a different browser and/or a different computer the server will not "recognize" you.

Web sites can store more than just one's ID, however. What they actually store is a combination of an item name (i.e., "user ID") and a value for that item (i.e., "123xyz"). A site can store several such pairs of item name-item values. For example, certain sites (such as Yahoo) allow a user to develop a customized home page (My Yahoo) with content pertaining to their geographic area, news preferences, and web page appearance. The display could be generated using cookies such as the following set:

YahooID	123xyz
YahooZip	19001
YahooNews	InternatUSSport
YahooColors	BlueGreen

Cookie data moves along the following pathway. When a user tells a browser to contact a web site (server) the browser checks its store of cookies (i.e., the IE cookie folder on your drive called Temporary

Internet Files) to see if there is a corresponding cookie file there. If so, it sends the cookie to the server along with the request for its web page. The server receives the cookie and the web page request and uses the cookie appropriately, in most cases to determine if the user has visited before (through a look-up in its table of known user ID's). If the user is known, the web site may tailor the returned web page to that user. For example, Amazon will display a list of recommended books based both on a known user's previous purchases and sophisticated software that tracks the reading patterns of all of its customers. If the user is unknown, the server will generate a new user ID and send it back with the requested web page.

The server may also change the value of a cookie stored on a user's machine. For example, if the Yahoo user referred to in the previous paragraph moved to a different zip code, he might change his Yahoo "home" page preferences, and the Yahoo server would change cookies on his computer accordingly to read:

YahooID	123xyz
YahooZip	19999

Cookies can also store information as to when they expire, when they were last changed, as well as several other pieces of standard data. In fact, a cookie has six elements including its name, the value associated with the name, its expiration date, the path the cookie is valid for, the domain the cookie is valid for, and whether or not the is intended only for secure connections (i.e., for banking or commercial interactions). The expiration value can be set for some time in the future or left blank, in which case the cookie expires at the conclusion of the user-browser interaction (Fig. 6-14).

Set-cookie:	
NAME = *VALUE*;	name of the cookie
expires = *DATE*;	how long it is valid
path = *PATH*;	where it is valid within a web site
domain = *DOMAIN_NAME*;	which domain (i.e. .com) it refers to
secure	whether or not is is secure

Figure 6-14
Cookies are used by servers to maintain continuity during successive client-server interactions.

Cookies were developed to solve a problem confronted by early web site developers: they had no way to store information about the users who visited the site. The fact that a web site can identify a specific user, even anonymously through that user's cookie-based ID, permits it to gather statistics about (1) how many visitors it sees, (2) how many of those visitors are new and how many have been to the site previously, and (3) how often a given visitor comes to the site.

Commerce sites can use the ID to implement features like the "shopping cart," in which the site keeps track of the items you intend to purchase during a given transaction with the web site by storing your cookie-derived ID with those items in a temporary database. When it is time to "check out," the web site retrieves everything you've identified for purchase from its temporary store, then prepares charge you and arrange shipping (Fig. 6-15).

It is probably worth revisiting some of the privacy issues that have been raised about cookies and their use. A safe, general statement is that the user has control over the cookies stored on his computer, unlike, for example, the actions of viruses and things like spyware. There are two issues that have raised privacy concerns about cookies. The first is the fact that by tracking what a user does on a given web site, the site's owner can then develop a profile of that specific user, in much the same way that mail order companies and supermarkets do. In addition, if that site has access to the user's email or actual address, it can use or sell that profile to others for targeted pitches.

These concerns were magnified when companies like DoubleClick, which tracks Internet usage on a large number of sites, developed the capability of creating rich, detailed, nonanonymous profiles of Internet users by following a user as he browsed across a number of sites (Fig. 6-16). In response to widespread concerns, DoubleClick implemented comprehensive, published privacy standards.

Users can control the cookies they get in a number of ways. The easiest, but the most constraining, is to reject all cookies. All browsers, but more specifically the Netscape and Microsoft versions, permit the user to control the handling of cookies either by selective filtering or nondiscriminatory rejection. In the latest versions of IE, the user can filter cookies by source and based on whether or not there is a privacy policy associated with that source. There is also the option to be warned before accepting a given cookie (Fig 6-17).

While a more draconian solution, one can choose to delete the entire cookie file, which will protect privacy, although it will mean that you "start from scratch" with every web site you visit thereafter. Many web sites have eliminated this problem through the use of login procedures whereby one explicitly logs on to the web site to identify oneself, rather than presenting identification information in the form of a cookie.

Popups and Popunders

There are a variety of programming tricks that use techniques to permit the browser to perform actions that the user may not have requested, such as opening a new window or windows unilaterally. Popups are windows that open on top of the requested window, often lacking many of the toolbar controls of a normal browser window. Popunders are essentially the same thing except that they open under the requested window and become visible only when the user moves or closes the original browser window.

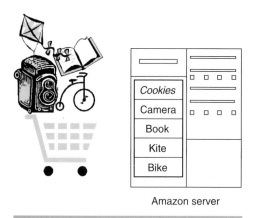

Figure 6-15
Cookies are often used by a web site to keep track of the items a user wishes to purchase as he "shops."

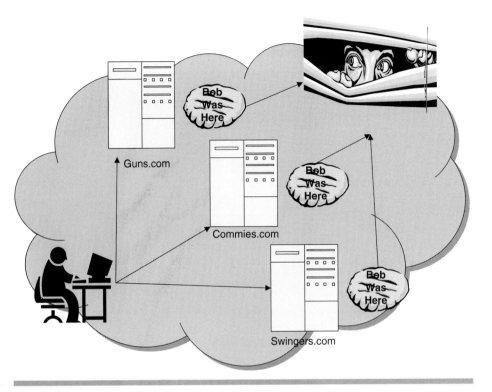

Figure 6-16
Cookies can be used to keep track of the sites a person visits.

Popups and unders can be useful. Some sites, for example, will "popup" a window permitting the user to click through the process of accepting the risks associated with downloading software from a vendor. Once the "I accept" button is clicked, the popup closes and the user proceeds to download the desired software product.

These features have been widely abused, however, at some sites to open a series of windows featuring advertisements or other undesirable content. AOL uses popups extensively to make advertising pitches or to handle browsing on the site. In some cases, the attempt to close the popup spawns a whole series of new offspring windows.

A ubiquitous, and apparently quite effective, popunder was the advertisement for the X10 wireless video camera. The advertisements were almost omnipresent during a period, and data captured at one point showed that the company reached 33% of the entire Internet's audience between January and May 2001, making it the fourth most visited site behind AOL, Microsoft, and Yahoo. On the other hand, while many visitors arrived at the site, they often left in something less than 20 s and without having purchased the X10 (Fig. 6-18).

Pop windows use Javascript functions to control their display, form, and function. The "call" to open a pop window is inserted in the HTML code for the initially requested web page, and is in the form *window.open (url, windowName, features)*. This may seem a little obscure, but this little piece of computer code will open a window from the requested address (*url* = uniform resource locator), give it the assigned *windowName*, and control its features. The available *features* include the location in which the window opens, its size, what browser buttons (i.e., backward/forward) and menu buttons (i.e., file/edit/view) are shown, and window controls (i.e., scrollbars/resize).

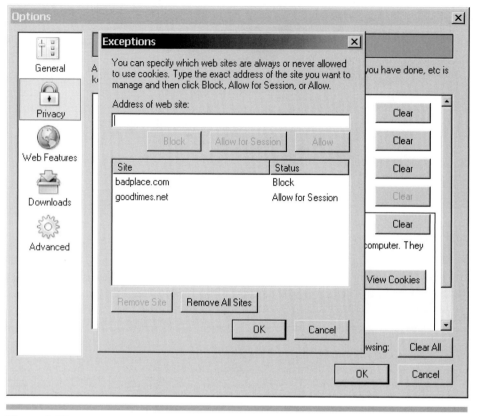

Figure 6-17
A user can block cookies from all or specific sites with most browsers.

While the X10 ads were effective initially, they quickly became annoying and widely reviled. As with many Internet pests which are developed by clever programmers, equally clever folks develop a response. Popup and under *blockers* prevent the display of these windows and are available for a fee from vendors or at no cost from Google and Yahoo. Pop blockers come in a variety of flavors. One way of preventing popups is to define "restricted sites," wherein Javascript applications are selectively disabled based on the originating address. Other approaches include intelligent popup killers, which attempt to distinguish between good and bad pop windows, trainable popup killers, which learn, with the user's feedback, which windows to reject, and browsers equipped with the ability to block popups. The Google and Yahoo pop blockers are useful in that they integrate with the primary browser to block unwanted windows (Fig. 6-19).

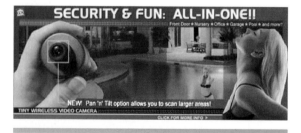

Figure 6-18
The X10 "popunder" was one of the first of what later became a wave of tools used to display unrequested advertisements on a user's PC.

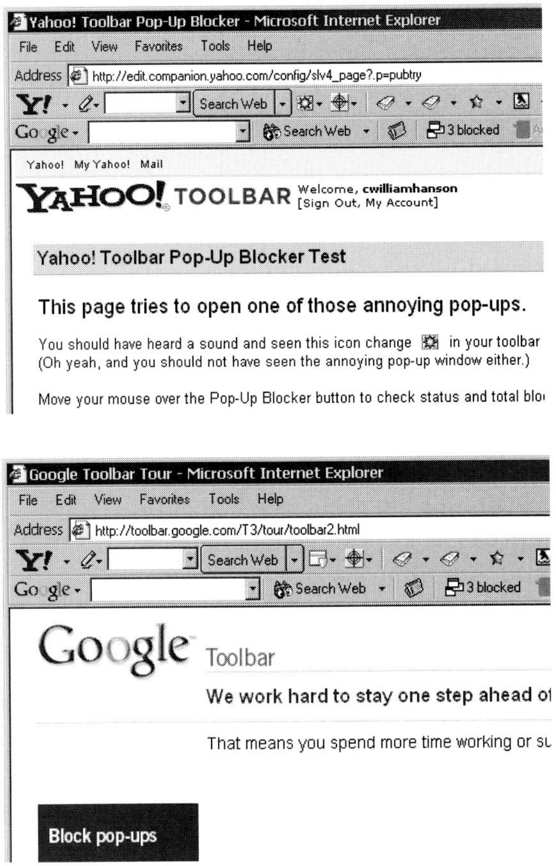

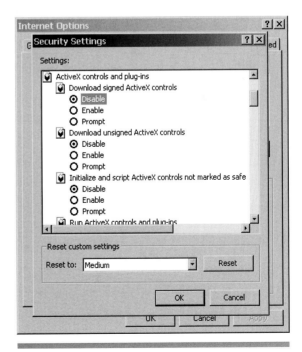

Figure 6-19
Web content providers responded to the wave of popups and popunders by developing popup "blockers."

Browser Safety

The browser is the computer user's window on the Internet, and for a long time it was safe to think of that window as being made of one-way glass. The user could choose to open the window and communicate through it, but only at his discretion.

It has become increasingly apparent that assumptions that were once safe are no longer so. Vulnerabilities in implementations of ActiveX, for example (Fig. 6-20), make it possible for malicious code to hijack control of the user's computer (causing the modem to dial charge by the minute

phone numbers, for example). Other malicious programs have been designed to watch activities of the user by logging keystrokes (and potentially storing passwords to web sites).

It is easy to create a "false front" web site that fools the unwary into thinking they are visiting a legitimate site, while the site is actually stealing the visitor's sensitive financial information. False front web sites that appear identical to the layout of sites such as AOL or Yahoo have been reported in the past. Finally, there are a number of other ways in which malicious code can be used to steal secure information from the unwary user.

Secure Browser Communications

Key Points

- Browsers are able to communicate securely with web servers permitting safe commercial and secure communications over the Internet.

Figure 6-20
Many users disabled Active-X controls as it became apparent that they could be designed to act unsafely by malicious programmers.

■ Browsers and servers verify each other's credentials, agree on a cipher (code) to use, and then communicate using coded interactions.

Browser security is clearly essential to communications over the Internet, and is used for interactions with web-based vendors, banks, and other sensitive communications. There are a variety of approaches to secure Internet communications, but the one used in most browsers is called secure sockets layer (or SSL), which was built into the early Netscape browsers.

The process involves three major components: a request for secure communication, a software "handshake" agreement between the browser and the server, and the establishment of a secure connection between the browser and the server, also known as a pipe. The request for secure communication occurs when the user browses to a site whose address begins "https", as opposed to the traditional "http." The "s" indicates that the server is providing secured communications. The handshake agreement consists of a first step wherein the seller's server presents a token (public key) to the browser indicating that it is a registered secure services provider, as designated by a "certificate authority" such as a company called VeriSign (Fig. 6-21).

A certificate authority is a trusted third party to a transaction, which issues tamper proof digital "passports" authenticating the holder. The browser contacts the server, which responds by sending its certificate indicating that it is who it says it is. This is followed by a second step in which the browser and server agree on how securely (how many bits will be used) to encrypt communications (most browsers now use 128 bits). Finally, the browser and server establish a virtual communications "pipeline," consisting of hardware and software components, through which they channel their communications.

Assuming the foregoing steps are completed, the information traveling through the pipeline is as secure as the encryption protocol used for communications. While a full description of encryption techniques and issues is not within the scope of this chapter (see Chap. 7), suffice it to say that one of the items agreed upon by the browser and

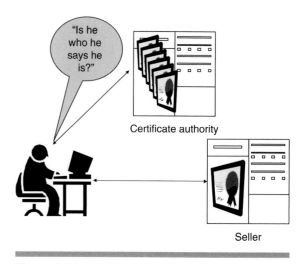

"Is he who he says he is?"

Certificate authority

Seller

Figure 6-21
Browsers can verify the credentials of a seller using the services of a trusted certificate authority.

the secure server is the cipher to be used for the session. There are a variety of ciphers available to SSL, and they vary in their strength, efficiency, and the degree to which the U.S. government permits their use. Some strong encryption approaches are not eligible for export, while others are restricted to use by government agencies.

Summary

One way to think of a browser is as a utility knife for your computer. The simplest browser needs only to be able to understand and display html documents, and that was essentially what the first browsers did. As the number of applications that a user might want to undertake on the Internet (i.e., hear sound, see animation, watch video clip) increased, the sophistication (read number of blades) of the browser "utility knife" has increased.

Suggested Readings

Smith BE, Bebak A. *Creating Web Pages for Dummies*, 6th ed. For Dummies, 2002.
http://www.pepmint.com/tutorial/index.html
http://www.supportcave.com/browsers.html

7 Security

 ## Introduction

Security is an ever-increasing concern for computer users and a critical issue for the medical community. Patient confidentiality is inherent to ethical medical care and the recent Health Insurance Portability and Accountability Act (HIPAA) legislation has focused a spotlight on the vulnerability of electronic medical data. Security breaches can result from mistakes, curious hackers, and/or malicious intruders. Computers newly attached to the Internet are scanned for open "doors" within a matter of seconds by various automated hacker probes.

Computer viruses, worms, and attacks have evolved from what were originally pieces of software typically designed to do mischief to what are now (often) professionally designed programs with commercial or politically designed ends. The computer industry has effectively responded with its own "health care" system of companies whose sole purpose is computer "hygiene" or "treatment." There are companies that monitor the Internet for the emergence of new threats, companies that intentionally attack corporate information systems to reveal vulnerabilities and report them back to those corporations and companies that manufacture new software intended to create an "immune system" for computers and networks (Fig. 7-1).

The immune system analogy is a convenient way to think of computer security for a variety of reasons in that it provides a framework to discuss a number of different types of threats that are relevant to the healthcare environment. The individual computer can be dealt with as if it were a cell, while the health care system's network is the circulation and the Internet is the world at large.

 ## Computer Security

Key Points

- Keep passwords secure.
- Good passwords are hard to "discover" and easy to remember.
- "Viruses," "worms," and "Trojan horses" are different types of threats to individual computers.
- Antiviral software should be installed and definitions should be kept current to protect each PC attached (even intermittently) to a network.
- "Firewalls" inhibit threats arriving through network connections.

Computer logon is the way in which individuals identify themselves to a local machine and/or a network. The creation and maintenance of good passwords is critical to computer protection. Giving a password to a "friend" who can't logon can have bad consequences: actions taken with a computer logged in under someone's name are legally presumed to have been performed by that individual. Hackers work very hard to get passwords using techniques as primitive as "dumpster diving" and as sophisticated as so-called *dictionary attacks* where every word in the dictionary and common variants are used in attempts to break into a user's account (Fig. 7-2). While this sounds like an exhausting manual process, programs are available from the Internet that automate this attack. Good passwords use a combination of upper and lowercase letters, numbers, and symbols. They are long and typically have some underlying meaning to the password owner.

Computers are also commonly vulnerable to security breaches in the form of viruses, worms,

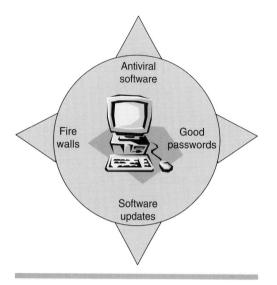

Figure 7-1
A computer can be made more secure through certain practices.

and so-called "Trojan horse" programs. Many people think of this kind of attack in conjunction with email, because most of the early forms of malicious code that spread from one computer to another came attached to email, and were activated when

an unsuspecting individual "opened" an file attached to email and thereby activated a program with a variety of consequences. Email attachments have been given the term "payload" in an analogy to the attack delivered by a bomb. Each of these attacks differs, however, in the way that it causes harm to a computer or a network. In order to give a sense of the magnitude of this problem, an industry standard email-monitoring program recently found that 1 in every 12 emails carried a virus or worm in 2004.

A computer virus attaches itself to an email or some other file (such as a picture downloaded from a website or a music file shared with someone over the Internet [Fig. 7-3]). The program comes along as a passenger and is not activated until the computer's user runs the virus program. Virus programs are programs that "run" when opened, and therefore have extensions that the operating system "understands" how to operate (i.e., ".exe" or ".bat"). A virus does not communicate itself from one computer to another automatically. As with real viruses, computer viruses come in a range of severities. A virus may do nothing more annoying that display a message, but may be malignant enough to disable a computer or erase memory.

Computer worms are similar to viruses insofar as they spread from one machine to another, but unlike viruses, they have the ability to travel without human intervention. Worms transmit themselves by using file or information transmission features built into an operating system such as the instant messaging system built into later versions

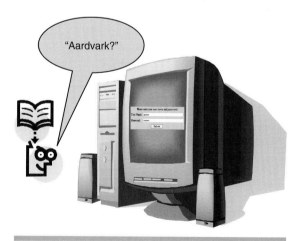

Figure 7-2
Hackers can "crack" easy passwords by systematically working their way through the dictionary.

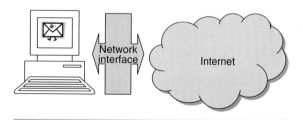

Figure 7-3
Computer viruses make their way on to a PC as attachments to email.

of Windows (Fig. 7-4). Worms also have the ability to replicate themselves on a single computer; one infected computer can therefore infect thousands of others. For example, a worm can infect a machine automatically, replicate itself, and send a copy to every email address listed on the infected computer and thereby create a cascade effect quickly affecting the entire Internet. The Sasser and Netsky worms are recent examples of programs that propagated very rapidly using a vulnerability in a component of the Windows operating system. The payload of variants of each of these worms was used to spread advertisements (Spam) automatically or attack specific websites, such as music file-sharing sites.

An additional undesirable feature inherent in worms is that they consume computer memory as they replicate or network bandwidth as they spread thereby "clogging up" the local machine or communications. As a result, individual computers or networks can perform slowly or stop altogether. Finally, some variants of recent worms have been used to allow remote users, such as Spammers, to take over individual computers and turn them into Spam creating "zombies." Note the commercial potential of automatic Spam generation programs—professional "worm writers," are paid for worms that generate Spam to buy an individual product, based on the degree to which sales increase or some other indicator of success. Spam represents an almost unbelievable 80% of all email in the first half of 2005.

Trojan horse software is named after the trick horse created by the Greeks to gain entry to Troy during the Trojan War. As with the horse, these programs appear to be attractive (i.e., screensavers) or useful (i.e., "Want to Remove Adware? Download This!") software provided for free on a website (Fig. 7-5). One recent Trojan horse program masqueraded as a Microsoft security update, whereas it actually disabled antivirus and/or firewall software. Trojan variants have deleted critical files and destroyed information on individual machines. Trojan horse programs do not self-replicate nor do they infect other files.

There are a variety of good general rules that one can follow to limit the chance of being affected by one of these problems. The first is never open an email attachment from an unknown individual. Because worms use email address books, it is possible that a person known to you may "send" an attachment that was actually generated by a self-replicating worm; therefore, a second rule is that you should never open an attachment from a known individual unless you know what the attachment contains.

Because computer attacks have become increasingly sophisticated (as with human viruses) and therefore able to elude defenses, it is essential to purchase and maintain antiviral software and keep the virus definitions up-to-date. Most good programs update themselves automatically using virus definitions maintained by companies that have an interest in keeping "up-to-the-minute" information from 24-hour command centers. Antiviral software programs typically also automatically scan any files arriving by email or downloaded from the Internet. These programs can and should be used to

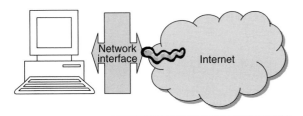

Figure 7-4
Computer worms propagate through "holes" in the software on a computer without any requirement for a user action (such as opening an email).

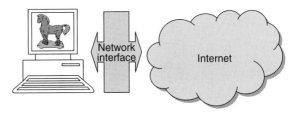

Figure 7-5
Trojan horse code is activated when a user does something (like download software from the web) that appears to be desirable but isn't.

scan a local system, such as system memory and attached hard drives on a regular basis (Fig. 7-6).

Another critical approach to protecting an individual machine is to download and install all operating system up-dates. Windows operating systems are claimed by some to be inherently vulnerable because they are poorly written, other believe that Microsoft is a particular target because of its size and dominance. The fact that Windows software is not "open-source," and that its vulnerabilities are less likely to be spotted than those of an operating system such as Unix may contribute as well. In any case, software patches issued by the vendor are intended to eliminate known vulnerabilities exploited by virus and worm writers and should be installed as quickly as possible. The cycle time between the identification of a problem and the release of a virus or worm that exploits that problem has become very short. Newer versions of Windows automatically update themselves with the user's permission (Fig. 7-7).

The final step in protecting an individual computer is the installation of a local firewall. As with a real firewall, a computer firewall is intended to slow or eliminate threats coming from outside of a protected environment. As part of the communications interaction with a network, every computer has a large number (greater than 65K) of "ports," i.e., windows and doors that it can open for communications. The first thousand are what are called "well-known ports." For example, there are specific port numbers for email communications, web page access, and file sharing.

Hostile intruders, like burglars, can conceptually test each of those ports to see if they are open and attack through them. While this kind of attack required a high degree of sophistication in the past, a novice hacker can now download automatic port-scanning software from the Internet and begin to scan computers across the Internet in a matter of minutes. Firewalls are designed to prevent attacks of this kind while still permitting legitimate bidirectional computer traffic (Fig. 7-8).

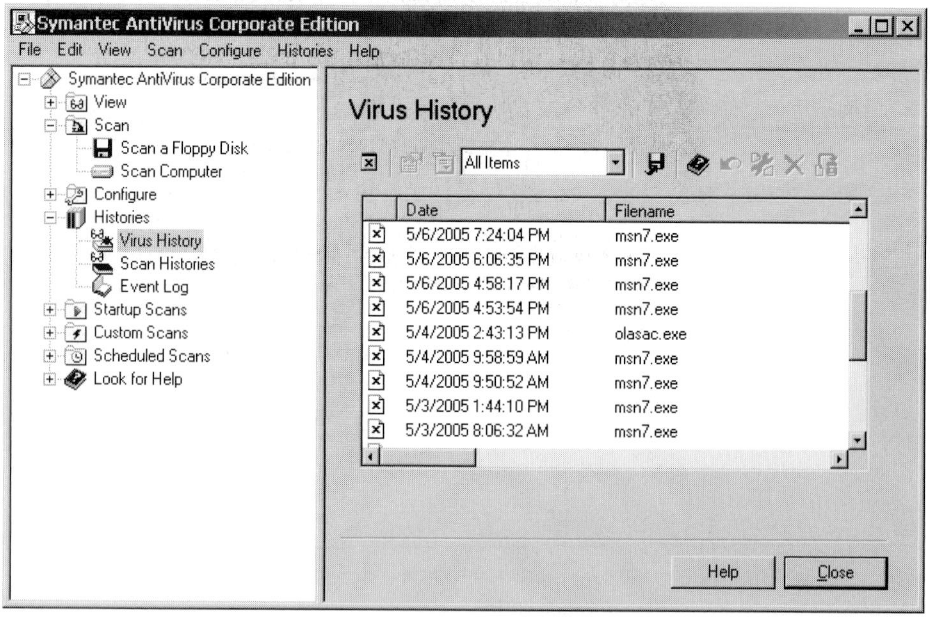

Figure 7-6
Antiviral software identifies and "quarantines" malicious software.

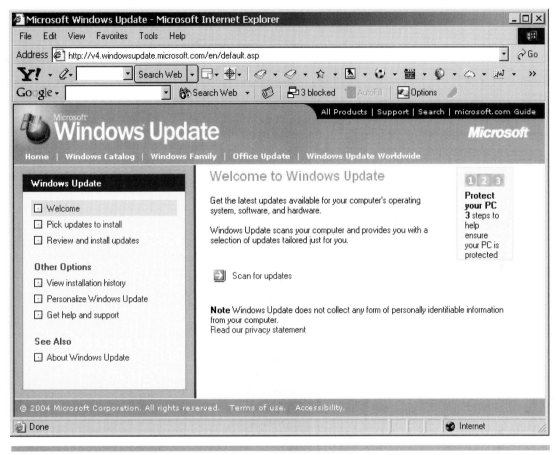

Figure 7-7
The user can close "holes" in software by applying patches or updates released by vendors.

Firewalls come in two general varieties. Hardware firewalls provide very good protection for some kinds of attacks but are less good than software

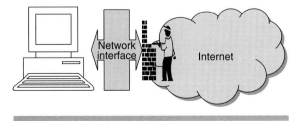

Figure 7-8
Computer firewalls prevent hackers from attacking through network interfaces.

firewalls at stopping others. A software firewall, for example, may recognize an embedded worm in an email because it has been specifically directed to look for it (via a virus definition update), whereas the hardware firewall might see that same email as legitimate. On the other hand, a hardware firewall may be far more efficient at screening traffic without slowing performance.

Hardware firewalls efficiently (quickly) look at each packet coming in from a network to determine where it came from (i.e., intranet vs. Internet) and where it's going and then decides whether to pass it on or drop it. More sophisticated versions look at issues such as whether or not the incoming traffic has a relationship to existing outgoing connections as with a webpage dialogue. Hardware firewalls don't block outgoing traffic very well if at all. This leaves open the possibility that an infected local machine might send out malicious packets such as Spam or sensitive information acquired from keystroke logging (wherein a malicious program keeps track of every keyboard stroke).

Software firewalls, on the other hand, can be told which programs are allowed to communicate over the network and over which ports. For example, by telling a software firewall that your designated email program is the only one allowed to use the email port, you could prevent a worm like the recent SoBig worm from using the same port to replicate from your machine.

Most home computers use software firewalls, and some newer operating systems, such as Windows XP, can be equipped without additional expense with a software firewall. Small home networks can be protected with hardware router firewalls that provide protection for more than one computer at their common point of attachment to the network. The exception is home networks using wireless connections, in which case additional wireless firewall protection is necessary.

■ Network Security

Key Points

- Threats to a network can come from within or without and may be malicious or inadvertent.
- For comprehensive protection, a variety of measures must be undertaken including human engineering as well as hardware and software measures.
- Sensitive medical information is much more susceptible to misuse in the age of computerization.
- Phishing is a modern version of old-fashioned fraud.
- Malware can infect a computer and degrade its performance as well as divert information to malicious programmers.
- It is possible to systematically attack a (hospital) network and degrade its performance or disable it.

The typical hospital information system has sophisticated security measures built into it, particularly since the passage of the HIPAA legislation described in Chap. 15. The corporate network is the distribution mechanism for many of the threats to computer security, and as with the human, networks employ a variety of immune mechanisms to protect the network (and its downstream users, the individual PCs) from threats. The first layer of defense is the network (as opposed to the PC) firewall. In this case, the firewall is a dedicated computer that runs special software monitoring both incoming and outgoing traffic. It can block certain types of traffic from passage. The corporate firewall and proxy server are often the same thing and act as an umbilical point at which IS department can control aspects of the hospital systems connection to the Internet (Fig. 7-9).

There is a tension between the desires of computer users and the administrators who run the Internet. While the goals of both are often aligned, security issues may be a point of departure. Users want easy and fast access to the Internet, whereas administrators want to keep the network secure. Network-specific security threats can be internal or external.

Internal Threats

Some of the potential internal threats into a hospital information system are discussed in Chap. 15. They include employees who attempt to steal or alter data, introduce viruses, or in some other way

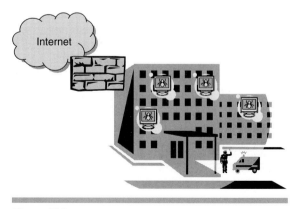

Figure 7-9
A hospital's information technology personnel will typically install and maintain antiviral software, software updates, and firewalls.

attack the network. Conversely, intruders may try to masquerade as an employee and perform the same bad actions. However, most internal threats are accidental, such as the employee who inadvertently releases a virus onto the network or downloads malware (see below) onto a nursing unit workstation.

Similarly employees may download or install personal software onto a workstation with unintended consequences to the computer's or network's performance. For example, an employee could load a game onto a workstation and thereby inadvertently release a virus or worm, or install poorly written or noncompliant software that cause the machine to fail.

The installation of unapproved hardware onto network machines is a major potential security breach. Modems and wireless access points that haven't been secured can provide an entryway for hackers or malicious software or an unsecured departure point for sensitive data. For example, sensitive medical data passing over an unauthorized wireless network within a medical setting could be picked up by someone "cruising" the street in a vehicle equipped with a wireless system (Fig. 7-10).

The term "war dialing" originated in a 1980s era movie about a teenage hacker who "dials in" to a military network, and modern era hackers have extended the term to "war driving." The term is now used to characterize the act of actively looking for open, unsecured wireless networks in a given geographic area. Just to give a sense of how problematic this may be, according to a recent study, 21% of home WiFi users can access their neighbors' wireless networks, and as many as 4% have "accidentally" logged on to those neighbor's systems, sometimes peeking at files and surfing the Internet through their broadband connection.

Unauthorized, portable storage and printing devices are another form of potential internal threat. A laptop plugged into a hospital network could be used to acquire sensitive medical data and transport it off site. Moreover, the development of high capacity portable universal serial bus (USB) drives has lowered the barrier to information removal even further. It is now possible to walk out of a hospital with gigabytes of sensitive data on a keychain (Fig. 7-11).

External Threats

External threats are varied and include threats inherent in the operating system or systems used in a hospital information system (HIS). These include email-related problems, interaction with malicious websites, instant messaging threats, a variety of file-sharing issues, and remote access vulnerabilities. The operating system threats have already been described and it is probably sufficient to add that more than 15,000 separate exploitable code vulnerabilities were reported in the last decade.

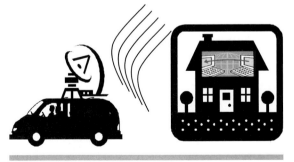

Figure 7-10
Some malicious users drive through neighborhoods with vehicles that scan for open wireless networks (so-called "war-driving") and then use them to access the Internet in the guise of the network's owner.

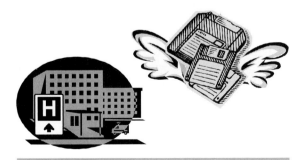

Figure 7-11
Confidential medical information is easily removed from a hospital using today's high-capacity electronic storage media.

Some relate to the correct performance of good code, analogous to breakable windows in a house, and others to coding errors. Configuration errors are another potential problem, such as the failure to assign a password to a computer when it first arrives, analogous to the failure to lock the door to your house.

Network communications are vulnerable to an approach called "packet sniffing," wherein a program intercepts network traffic between two sites looking at the address on each packet. By copying all packets with a specific address, a fragmented series of packets can be reconstructed into a coherent communication such as a file or email. There are a variety of other ways in which to intercept network traffic, and surveillance products are readily available on the Internet for casual hackers (Fig. 7-12).

Some of the varied email attacks have been described above and in the chapter on email. In addition to viruses, email can arrive with embedded scripts and webpage controls that can cause unwanted actions by a computer. Alternatively, email can contain attached webpage links that, when clicked, take the user to a web page with malicious code that can run by itself.

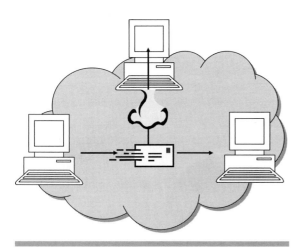

Figure 7-12
Malicious parties can tap into traffic crossing the Internet ("packet sniffing") and thereby gain access to confidential communications.

Phishing

A newly emerging email threat is what is known as *phishing*, whereby fraudulent email messages seemingly sent from legitimate sites (i.e., eBay) are used to attempt to convince recipients to divulge passwords, social security numbers, credit card numbers, or other sensitive data (Fig. 7-13).

Employees may be promoted to download malicious software, download illegal files (such as copyrighted music) putting the organization at risk or install pirated software in a network. Each of these activities represents a separate externally originating threat to a system.

Systematic Network Attacks

Finally, it is possible to attack a network using any of hundreds of different techniques. The network can be degraded or brought to a stop using methods such as denial of service (DOS) attacks in which a system is flooded with malicious messages or data to the point that legitimate network traffic is brought to a stop. Distributed DOS attacks occur when a large number of computers are conscripted (by worms, for example) and turned into zombies that can simultaneously attack a network or computer, making it impossible to point to the origin of the attack (Fig. 7-14).

Malware

Malware is a generic term referring to software products that behave badly on one's computer. The term is used to comprehensively describe malicious software, such as adware, spyware, or page hijackers (described below).

Adware   Adware is any software application responsible for the display of advertising on a user's computer. The authors of these applications create programs that deliver the ads, which can be viewed through popup windows or through a bar that appears on a computer screen. Adware may include program code that can be used to track a user's personal information and pass it on to third parties without the user's authorization or knowledge. Adware may be legitimate software, or it

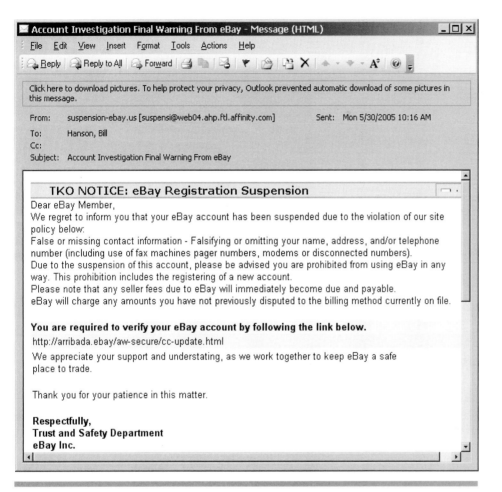

Figure 7-13
"Phishing" is designed to lure unwary individuals into revealing confidential information using techniques like this phony notice.

may be a separate program that is unknowingly installed with another downloaded or purchased program. Not all adware is bad, but often users are annoyed by adware's intrusive behavior. Often adware makers make their application difficult to uninstall.

Spyware   Spyware is more dangerous than adware because it can record your keystrokes, surfing history, passwords, and other confidential and private information. Spyware may be explicitly sold as a "spouse monitor", "child monitor", and surveillance tool or as a tool to spy on users to gain unauthorized access. Spyware covertly gathers user information and activity without the user's knowledge and can record keystrokes as they are typed, including passwords, credit card numbers, visited web sites, chat logs, or take random screenshots. This spying can occur while a user is on the web or information can be stored and surreptitiously send elsewhere when the user connects to the web.

Many spyware programmers use techniques to avoid detection and removal by popular antispy software including routines to reinstall the

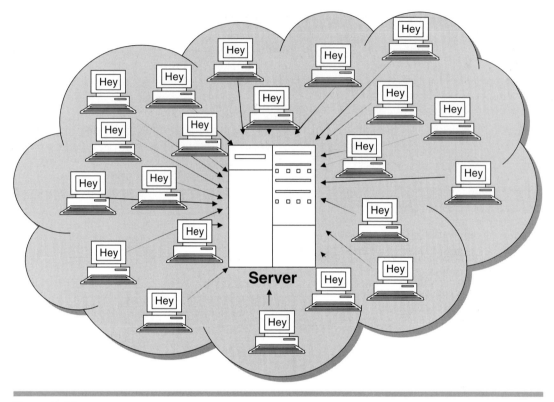

Figure 7-14
"Denial of service" attacks are intended to overwhelm a server or system with incoming traffic, often from PCs that have been infected with a virus designed to coopt them for this purpose.

spyware application after it has been detected and supposedly deleted.

Page Hijackers Hijackers are programs that attempt to take control of the user's preferred home page and replace it with one of the hijackers choosing. Search hijackers replace one's default search engine. As a result, undesirable advertisements and advertising contents are "found" rather than relevant search results.

Dialers

A dialer is a type of software often used by pornographic vendors. Once dialer software is downloaded the user is disconnected from their modem's usual Internet service provider and another long

distance phone number is called and the user is billed. While dialers do not spy on users they are malevolent in nature because they can cause huge financial harm to the victim.

RATs

Remote administration tools (RATs) are designed to allow an attacker to gain unrestricted access to a user's computer. The attacker can thereby perform activities such as file transfers, adding/deleting files or programs, and controlling the mouse and keyboard.

Malware Consequences

There are several signs suggesting that a computer is "infected" with some form of malware, including the display of malware when a computer is not online. Alternatively, the browser starts up with an unrecognized home page, new browser toolbars, slowed performance, or computer crashes as a result. Computers may suddenly popup pornographic material or slow to the point that they become unusable. Fortunately, a number of anti-malware products have recently been released for no charge from companies such as Yahoo, Microsoft, and Lavasoft (Ad-aware). These products maintain up-to-date information about existing threats and can be used both to scan a computer and clean it of known malware.

VPN Vulnerabilities

The ability to access an HIS from a remote location is increasingly critical to the ordinary course of doing business. Remote practitioners may need to gain access to medical information from locations that aren't hardwired into the intranet. Employees may need to have access to data from within the network when traveling. Dial-up access into a remote access server is an increasingly dated paradigm. More typically, networks now provide a virtual private network server. There are special and unusual risks that relate to simultaneous broadband and VPN connections. For example, a user attached to the Internet using a hotel broadband connection might have simultaneously connected to the HIS VPN servers through a modem on the same laptop. This is called split tunneling and presents a potential security risk.

Summary: Consequences

Security breaches have been romanticized in movies such as Hackers and War Games, but the consequences to patients, clinicians, and health systems can be significant. Individuals whose personal computers are breached can suffer consequences such as identity theft, intrusion into private email "conversations," and the loss or alteration of data files. It is even possible for a malicious hacker to "plant" pornographic or other information on a machine with criminal ramifications for the unwitting victim.

Viruses and other malware can have damaging effects on network performance. One estimate put the cost of an *hour* of downtime in a healthcare setting at roughly $100K. It is difficult to evaluate the potential for direct healthcare consequences for individual patients although these will become more apparent as the industry becomes more reliant on computer systems for information transmission and decision support.

There are a number of other more intangible costs, such as the labor and materials to detect and repair damage to individual computers as when viruses propagated within an intranet. Worker productivity is diminished when they must resort to backup systems. The HIPAA legislation permits both fines and jail sentences for individuals who knowingly release protected health information. A health system can also be subjected to penalties for security breaches if it is shown to be noncompliant with HIPAA or other computer regulatory standards.

Suggested Readings

Greene TC. *Computer Security for the Home and Small Office*. Apress, 2004.

Rothke B. *Computer Security: 20 Things Every Employee Should Know*. Osbourne: McGraw-Hill, 2003.

Pfleeger CP, Pfleeger SL. *Security in Computing*, 3rd ed. New York: Prentice-Hall, 2002.

Hospital Information Systems

Introduction: History of the HIS

Key Points

- Hospital information systems (HISs) started as business, financially oriented systems rather than patient-care-oriented, clinical systems.

- While the potential promise of artificial intelligence was clear from the outset, despite some successful demonstration projects, they never took hold in patient care.

- The fundamental principles for the design of good medical computer systems have changed since they were first described in the 1960s.

- Early medical systems were deployed on "mainframe" computers and interfaced to the user through "dumb" terminals.

- As clinical subsystems (i.e., radiology) were developed and matured, many hospitals took a "best-in-breed" approach and married disparate systems to one another through a central hub.

- The alternative approach is to go to a core vendor who supplies most of the needed services.

Hospitals were a logical and early spot for the implementation of computerized processes. The history of hospital information systems goes back to the 1960s and the early players included IBM and a company known at the time as Burroughs (which subsequently merged with Sperry Rand to become what is most recently known as Unisys). There were also a number of smaller, medical software companies that originated in the 1960s and 70s such as IDX, Shared Medical Systems (which is now owned by Siemens), and Meditech. These companies were all focused on patient billing (Fig. 8-1).

As is the way with all industries, the medical software industry has undergone substantial consolidation and reformation over the past 3–4 decades, but it is still possible to discern the evolution of the requirements that drove the development of the hospital information system of today.

The possibilities of medical computing were recognized in the very early days of computing, and artificial intelligence applications were developed very early for medicine. Articles can be found dating back to the end of the 1950s pertaining to the potential applications of medical electronics. Certain medical institutions and individuals developed medically oriented computing programs in the 1960s and early 1970s, such as Octo Barnett M.D. at MGH who led the development of the MUMPS programming language, which was designed for medical computing applications. Patient screening and health evaluation programs were developed at Kaiser Permanente in California and the Latter Day Saints hospital in Salt Lake City. Medline, the on-line version of the Index Medicus, was developed in the early 1960s. There were other clinically oriented projects, but it was really patient billing that drove the corporate development of medical software.

Octo Barnett developed a set of commandments, many of which are fundamentally applicable to today's health care informatics environment:

1. Thou shall know what you want to do (i.e., be clear-cut in your design goals).

2. Thou shall construct modular systems (i.e., develop computer programs as constructs of

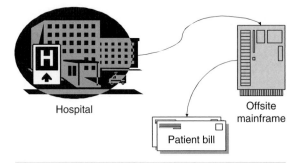

Figure 8-1
The first hospital computers were designed for patient billing and were often owned by off-site contractees.

interlocking parts so that you can update and repair readily).

3. Thou shall build a system that can evolve (i.e., and grow over time) in a graceful fashion.

4. Thou shall build a system that allows easy and rapid programming development and program modification (so that the barriers to modification are low).

5. Thou shall build a system that has a consistently rapid response time and is easy for the noncomputernik to use.

6. Thou shall have duplicate (redundant) hardware systems (i.e., so the system doesn't "go down" very often).

7. Thou shall build and implement systems as a joint effort with real users in a real situation with real problems (i.e., so clinicians will like and use the system rather than as the programmer thinks it should be designed).

8. Thou shall be concerned with the realities of the cost and projected benefit of the computer system.

9. Innovation in computer technology is not enough; there must be an equal commitment to the potentials of radical change in other aspects of health care delivery, particularly those having to do with organization and

manpower utilization (i.e., it makes no sense to computerize if delivery paradigms can't change at the same time).

10. Be optimistic about the future, supportive of good work that is being done, passionate about your commitment, but always guided by fundamental skepticism.

Mainframe Monolithic Systems

Billing systems were implemented on mainframe computers in programming languages designed for the management of patient "records" (such as COBOL: Common Business Oriented Language). In some cases the computers that performed the billing tasks were located off-site and multiple computers shared access to central computers over dedicated phone lines. Accurate information about the state of the hospital and the location of patients was a necessary adjunct to computerized billing, so the "admissions, discharge, transfer" (ADT) function was computerized early on as well (Fig. 8-2).

Larger hospitals developed in-house "data processing" departments with personnel dedicated to transcribing manual patient information onto punched cards, the transaction medium of the time. Punched cards were used in tabulating machines long before

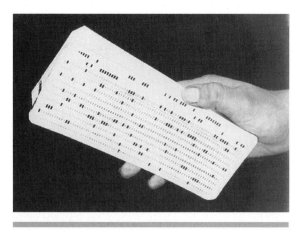

Figure 8-2
Data was entered using punched cards which were created by dedicated data entry personnel.

the development of computers, but became the major data storage mechanism for most computers until well into the 1970s. Both programs and data could be stored on these cards, which were rectangular cards in a preformatted layout. A hole punched in a given location represented a piece of data, such as a letter or number. Parenthetically, the small cardboard remnant from a punched hole is known as a chad. The punched card voting machine (Votomatic) that became so notorious during the 2000 (remember "hanging chad") presidential elections is one example of several similar techniques for storing data to be entered into a computer.

Modular (best-in-breed) Systems

The next major development in the area of hospital information systems came with the advent of modular computers dedicated to laboratory or radiology functions. Early laboratory products like Statlan reported lab information to clinical floors through video display terminals linked to dedicated, on-site mainframe computers. Information relating to patient identification and location was maintained on an ADT computer and relayed to lab, radiology, and pharmacy machines through customized interfaces.

The modular approach can be contrasted to the all-in-one approach (Fig. 8-3), where one company provided a comprehensive solution for all of a hospital's HIS needs. The modular approach allowed a customer to select the "best-in-breed" solution for each module, but suffered from the need to develop customized interfaces between the modules and difficulties in integration. With the modular best-in-breed approach, each vendor had preferred, usually mutually incompatible approaches to interfacing with other machines. Incompatibilities and the need for negotiation with two parties (the two vendors) put customers at a disadvantage and made for lengthy, costly development processes; and the resulting interfaces were fragile, complicated, and resource intensive.

With the advent of smaller machines, called microcomputers, primitive networking began to develop and we began to see the development of ward computers with local computer networks.

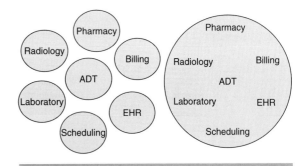

Figure 8-3
There are two general extremes of approaches to hospital information systems: "best-in-breed" systems (left) use the best vendor for each subsystem and marry them together while all-in-one systems (right) are offered by some vendors and provide global solutions.

Individual offices remained isolated and few provider offices or examination areas had linked computers.

This period marks the beginnings of what is now thought of as a clinical information system, where clinically oriented computers (such as laboratory or radiology systems) were linked to provider sites using "dumb" terminals. Toward the latter end of the 1980s, personal computers started to replace "dumb" video display terminals at service locations and come into widespread use as office management equipment in provider offices. Office-based PCs were linked to billing systems to centralize scheduling and billing. Private offices usually linked to central computers using modems and the phone system.

During the early part of the 1990s, many hospitals were wired with computer cable which marked the beginnings of hospital intranets. Personal computers began to be deployed at service locations, such as nursing stations, and the hospital intranets began to provide access to the Internet. Simultaneously, individual subsystems of the hospital information system became more sophisticated (Fig. 8-4).

For example, what had originally been simple ADT systems became more differentiated into separate registration and scheduling functions. Pharmacy systems grew more comprehensive and

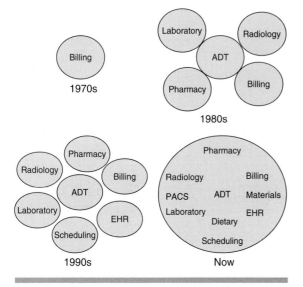

Figure 8-4
HISs have evolved in scope and complexity over the
past several decades.

developed drug monitoring and unit dosing components. Financial management programs, which were originally purely for patient billing, began to integrate management reporting tools for administrators.

The complexity and cost of medical computing grew exponentially after PCs and networks became widely deployed in the hospital setting.

Modern Health Information Systems

Key Points

- Modern health information systems (HISs) are complex, interwoven systems with many missions including the acquisition of information from patient (through direct interfaces to laboratory and radiology diagnostic equipment), the deliver of information to clinicians, and the management of the business of medicine.

- Communication among disparate subsystems requires the development of interfaces and common "languages."

- HL7 is an example of an industry standard messaging protocol, by which, every system has a

common understanding of what constitutes a medical record number, for example.

- Interface engines are an example of what is known as "middleware" in the computer industry, and designed to act as universal translators.

Over the last decade, hospital information systems have become complex meshes of interlocking and overlapping subcomponents. Front-end machines such as laboratory analyzers and radiographic scanners are computerized. Information from these machines is passed on to routing and processing machines and then to providers. In the case of radiographic information, for example, an original data set (i.e., CT scan) is acquired from the CT machine, sent on to an interpretation workstation where it is read by a radiologist, who may then dictate a report into an automated transcription machine. The image information and report are then married and made available for remote viewing by primary clinicians on a picture archiving and communica tions system (PACS). Finally, the image and report are stored for a period in a short-term archive before ultimate storage in a long-term archive (Fig. 8-5).

In addition to the clinical systems, modern health information systems have all of the components of a typical business system as well. It has file servers where users store their data documents, mail servers through which users send and receive e-mail, web servers that host the organization's web sites, database servers that store information in easily queried format and emote access, and/or VPN

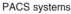

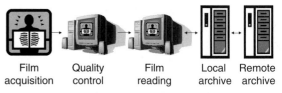

| Film acquisition | Quality control | Film reading | Local archive | Remote archive |

Figure 8-5
X-ray images pass through quality control computers, are read and then sent to local and eventually long-term archives from which they can be retrieved on request.

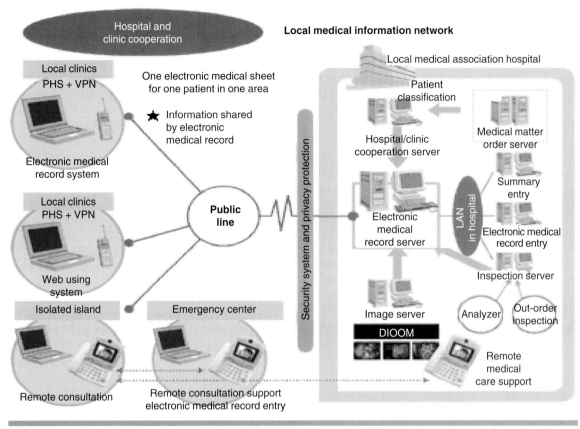

Figure 8-6
Modern HISs are likely to encompass a variety of geographically distinct sites and using public phone or digital networks.

servers through which employees and partners can connect to the LAN from home, while on the road, or from other remote sites. Network access is handled by authentication servers (domain controllers on Windows-based networks) that verify users' credentials to log on to the network (Fig. 8-6).

Complex hospital information systems have many subsystems, all of which need to communicate amongst themselves to varying degrees (Fig. 8-6). The old paradigm, in which customized, labor-intensive interfaces were built for each juncture point between computers, would be unmanageable in today's world. The customized interface has been replaced by an *interface engine* (Fig. 8-7).

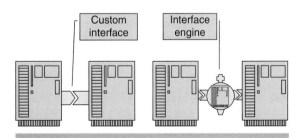

Figure 8-7
A custom interface is specifically tailored for communications between two computers, whereas an interface engine is a general-purpose communication link.

An interface engine sits in the conceptual center of a network taking incoming messages from one computer and translating them to the format desired by the destination computer before send them on. For example, a field called "medrecno," in which leading zeros are used to ensure that the data is 10 digits long may be reformatted to the "Medic_Record_Num" field required by a different computer which doesn't use leading zeros. Interface engines and the development of a standard set of rules for data exchange across systems were what permitted the development of today's large heterogeneous health information systems.

HL7

This standard, Health Level Seven which is usually called "HL7," is both an American National Standards Institute (ANSI)-accredited standards organization and a standard in and of itself. The organization was founded in 1987 with an original committee of 14 people. It now numbers nearly 2000 members including healthcare providers, vendors, and consultants (Fig. 8-8).

HL7 is an example of a defined set of rules about communications in computing called a protocol. A concise definition of a protocol is "a coordinated, message-based connection between two systems allowing information to be exchanged reliably between the systems." Some of the aspects of the

definition are as follows. "Coordinated" implies that the two systems know about the state of each other, where states could be "up," "down," "ready to receive," "not ready to receive," and so on. Message-based implies that there is an unambiguous, predefined structure to the data being exchanged, with which both systems are familiar. "Reliably" means that error-free delivery is guaranteed: delivery efforts are continued until they are successful, and the message is delivered intact (exactly as it was sent).

Custom Interfaces

Prior to the development of HL7, a custom built interface between two subsystems could cost anywhere from $50 to $250K, whereas the same interface today costs a fraction of that. These cost reductions are a function of the fact that HL7 has come to represent the standard used to determine what information (i.e., a new patient laboratory study) flows where (i.e., to a clinical information subsystem interested in that lab) and when (i.e., stat). The mission of the HL7 standards organization is to create standards that the healthcare software industry can use to facilitate the exchange, management, and integration of data supporting patient care and the management and delivery of healthcare services.

HL7 has grown from its initial inception in the late 1980s to an international consensus standard. While HL7 was initially designed for messaging across interfaces, it has evolved beyond that limited role. One major problem inherent in the coexistence of disparate systems is the disparity in their "look and feel." One system, for example, might have an old-fashioned command line interface (like Statlan), whereas another might have a slick, animated interface. Vendors have come to recognize that it is the interests of all to provide relatively seamless integration, as with Office software packages.

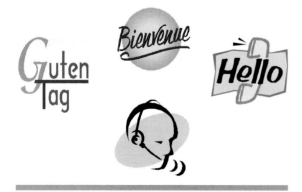

Figure 8-8
HL7 is the "universal language" of medical computing devices.

CCOW

The HL7 standards organization published the Clinical Context Management Specification (also known as CCOW) in 1999. This standard established a method to enable end-users to seamlessly view results from disparate "back-end" clinical systems as if they were integrated. This mutual interest standard is analogous to the standards used to ensure that every endotracheal tube (regardless of size or vendor) connects to every manufacturer's ventilator circuit (Fig. 8-9).

HL7 also published the Arden Syntax for medical logic in 1999, which is a language that can be used for the description and encoding of medical decision making. Arden is used as a standard to encode clinical reminders, alerts, lab interpretations and diagnoses.

Beyond the cost savings associated with using HL7-based interfaces, there is a savings in the time and effort it takes to design an interface between two machines. The amount of work needed to connect subsystems grows quickly with the number of subsystems, and in today's hospital information systems, there are likely to be a large and increasing number of individually tasked computer systems that need to communicate with one another. HL7 dramatically reduces the interface implementation time and efficiency.

It is probably correct to say that without the combination of HL7 and interface engines, today's hospital information systems would not be possible or would run so slowly that the performance would be unacceptable.

Interface and Integration Engines

An *interface engine* belongs to a class of software known in as "middleware," and is designed to relieve software applications from the responsibility of worrying about integration with other applications (i.e., the need to integrate an interface into the product). Middleware programs are also called "message brokers," and fall into one of two broad categories: interface engines and integration engines. Interface engines incorporate message definition and management tools and built-in support for standard and common protocols such as HL7, DICOM (Digital Images and Communications in Medicine: a radiographic image standard), and ASTM (American Society for Testing and Standards: a medical laboratory standard). An interface engine also guarantees message delivery.

An *integration engine* does somewhat more than an interface engine, but accomplishes essentially the same results. Without going into unnecessary detail, there are two general approaches that achieve the same results. In one the message broker accepts an incoming message (such as a notice of a patient discharge), validates it (ensures that it is formatted correctly), translates or reformats it (if necessary), and forward it to other computers in the hospital information system. The alternate approach is one in which the message broker validates the message, "publishes" it, and other computers on the system having an interest in messages of that sort "subscribe to" (read) them.

Message "Transactions" in an HIS

A typical transaction on a modern HIS involves a change in patient status such as a new admission. The new patient interacts with an admissions clerk who gathers relevant demographic and insurance information. This data is typed into the ADT system, which sends out a message on the network consisting of the data packaged in a precise format. The ADT system broadcasts the message

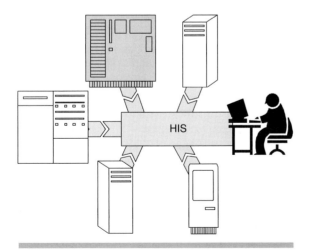

Figure 8-9
Modern HISs provide seamless integration among disparate systems using tools like interface engines and HL7.

with no preconceived notions about the systems that might receive the message (it doesn't really care), but with the expectation that it will receive an acknowledgement from somewhere that the message was accepted. It will not broadcast any more information without the acknowledgement. The interface engine receives the admission message, may or may not reformat it, and queues it for delivery to the systems that are interested in that information (such as the lab, pharmacy, or radiology systems) (Fig. 8-10).

The interface engine is configured to know about what systems are interested in what messages and what their current status is. The interface engine would know, for example, if the lab system was "down" for a period and continue attempting to deliver its admission message until it is successful.

The interface engine loosens the linkages between the component machines of a hospital information system in the same way that banks do financial transactions, which has the paradoxical effect of improving the integrity and reliability of these linkages. Take the act of using one's a credit card in a foreign country, for example. The credit card company acts as an intermediary between the foreign merchant and you the customer. It pays the merchant and you pay the credit card company, and the current exchange rate is applied by the credit card's bank. The company uses something like an exchange rate table to apply the current (and constantly changing) rate dur-

ing any such transaction. Similarly, prior to the development of interface engines, for example, a change in a medical data file specification (like an ICD9 code) would necessitate a costly and time consuming rewrite of the custom interface. Today, that same change is handled by the modification of a translational table in the interface engine (Fig. 8-11).

Credit card companies also act to ensure the integrity and reliability of a monetary transaction. Provided the merchant delivers on his end of the bargain, the credit card company guarantees that he'll get his money even in a phone transaction where he never sees the customer. Similarly, the interface engine guarantees delivery of a message, from a lab system to a nursing station computer for example, even if the nursing unit computer is "down" at the time of original message transmission.

Network Backbones

Another important advantage of the use of interface engines is the fact that, unlike traditional interfaces between two computers, where there is a one to one relationship, interface engines permit "one to many" transactions. In an older HIS, for example, an ADT computer would sit at the center, or hub, of a "spoke and wheel" network. It would have "one to one" interfaces (spokes) with each of the computers on the system. In today's architectures, there is a common communications "backbone," and component computers can attach at any point along the backbone (Fig. 8-12). In a typical transaction, the ADT computer, somewhere on the backbone, sends a new patient admission message to the interface engine elsewhere on the backbone.

The interface engine checks the integrity of the message and it may reformat the message. The message can then be stored or forwarded to other computers on the system in need of that information, such as the lab, pharmacy, or radiology computer systems.

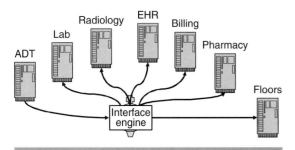

Figure 8-10
Typical transaction on an HIS might be the notification of a patient admission by the ADT system to the interface engine, which then broadcasts the message to all systems having an interest in patient location.

Conclusion

As medical software applications become more sophisticated, information coming from many

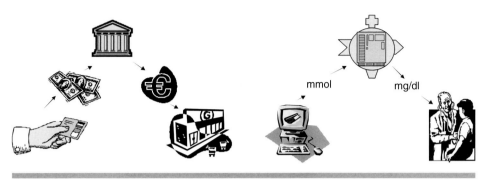

Figure 8-11
Banks maintain current exchange rates in dealing with various currencies in much the
same way that medical interface engines maintain current exchange tables.

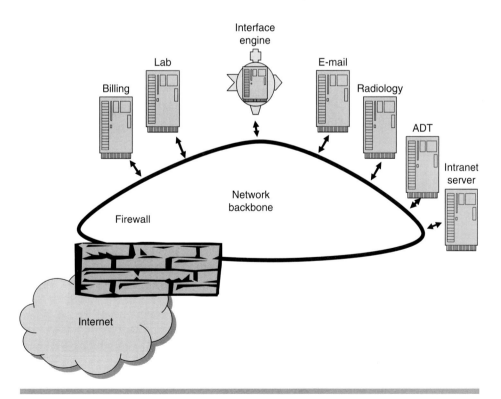

Figure 8-12
Modern networks are often configured as loops, which ensures that there are
redundant pathways between any two computers on the backbone.

sources is increasingly aggregated for display on a common software interface. There are many obvious advantages to this approach. The clinician doesn't have to sign on to many different systems, and need only sign on once. The clinician's interface is designed to aggregate all patient information for display through a single "portal."

An example of this approach is an electronic medical record (EMR) application in which the same screen may show patient location (derived from the ADT system), laboratory results (from the lab system), radiology results (from the radiology system), and medication information (from the pharmacy system). It is obviously essential to ensure that the information displayed on a given patient is as current as possible. One method is to have the EMR actively query the other systems (i.e., radiology) each time the clinician requests relevant data (i.e., an x-ray report). Alternatively, the interface engine can keep a copy of the entire record and maintain the necessary data fields. This releases the EMR from the burden of knowing information about the other computers and transfers that responsibility to the interface engine, which is already doing business with all of the other computers on the network.

Suggested Readings

Haux R, Winter A, Ammenwerth E, et al. *Strategic Information Management in Hospitals: An Introduction to Hospital Information Systems.* Springer, 2004.

Van de Velde R, Degoulet P. *Clinical Information Systems: A Component-Based Approach.* Springer, 2003.

Electronic Medical Record

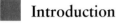

Introduction

Key Points

- The electronic medical record has been in development for 20 years, and will inevitably replace the paper record, but its adoption has been slow.

- Despite buy-in from the federal government, industry, and patient advocacy groups, the healthcare industry has lagged behind other industries in computerization of its records.

- Barriers include technical impediments, inadequate infrastructure, and the conservatism of the healthcare community.

- Electronic health records (EHRs) are now beginning to diffuse into the acute care health system and adoption is expected to increase rapidly in the next decade.

The electronic medical record will inevitably replace the paper record at some point in the near future. It has been the subject of extensive discussion and attention by industry and government; as of today, however, it remains a largely unrealized concept. The electronic record has been described variously as a computerized medical record, computerized patient record, electronic medical record, and more recently as an electronic health record (EHR). This last term will be used throughout this chapter (Fig. 9-1).

Any number of federal agencies, including the National Library of Medicine, the Agency for Healthcare Research and Quality, the Department of Defense, and the National Institute of Standards and Technology, as well as industry groups have attempted for over a decade to "jump-start" the development of computerized patient records. In spite of this EHRs are not used in most patient care settings. The technological barriers inherent in integrating EHRs into medical care are negligible compared to the human, behavioral, and organizational ones. Problems falling under the latter category include issues as fundamental as the definition of an EHR, the redefinition of the roles of the consumers of the medical record, and the creation of standards for data and data security (Fig. 9-2).

The barriers to the adoption of EHRs range from imperfect software and the lack of standards, to the cost of retooling. A recent Rand Corporation study found that 10–15% of the nation's office-based clinicians use EHRs in their practice, and that the speed of adoption is likely to increase rapidly as the technology improves and the cost of remaining paper-bound becomes increasingly apparent. In fact, some patients have taken the problem with traditional medical records into their own hands and subscribed to an on-line service permitting an individual to create their own "own-line" medical record.

The 2005 Rand study, entitled "The Diffusion and Value of Healthcare Information Technology" resulted in several key findings. The first is that, while later than many other industries, healthcare is slowly computerizing, and at a rate consistent with the other industries. EHRs are finally entering into the marketplace, and rapidly. Thirty percent of acute care hospitals had ordered EHR products at the conclusion of 2003; and, by 2016, 80% are expected to have computerized records.

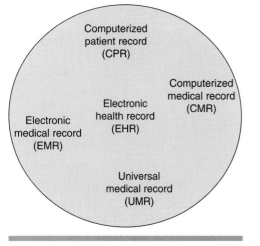

Figure 9-1
There are many equivalent names for a digital medical record.

Significant productivity increases can be expected in the medical industry, assuming EHRs are adopted and deployed effectively.

Paper Medical Record

Key Points

▇ The paper record is familiar and portable, but it can only be read by a single user at a single time, is formatted sequentially, and does not lend itself to the inclusion of alternative, non-paper-based content.

▇ Many first generation EHRs recreate the paper record and fail to take advantage of capabilities like hypertext-based browsing.

The paper medical record is a sequential record that is structured in a certain way due largely to historical precedents. Data are divided into different sections such as administrative, nursing, laboratory, and progress segments and most of the chart manipulation is done by clerks. The chart is limited to certain kinds of data entry; radiographic studies, for example, cannot be stored contiguously with progress notes (Table 9-1).

A clinician interested in the evolution of a specific problem area in the medical chart, such as

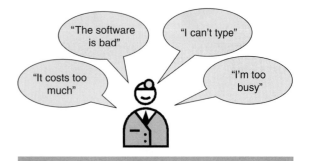

Figure 9-2
There are a variety of barriers to the adoption of medical records by health care practitioners.

renal failure, has to leaf through data pertaining to other problems. While these limitations are readily surmounted in an EHR, many industry-based implementations of electronic records recreate the paper-based record with its organization and limitations. Narrative rather than structured text documentation is common and there is limited ability to reformat or make use of tools such as hypertext. More advanced capabilities, such as multimedia, are not contemplated.

Electronic Health Record

Key Points

▇ The Institute of Medicine (IOM) convened a body of experts to describe the ideal EHR, which should provide an integrated view of patient data, as well as enhanced communication among providers, access to patient-specific educational content.

▇ The idea of an EHR dates back to the 1960s, at which time the problem-oriented medical record and computerized patient record keeping were

Table 9-1 Pros and Cons of the Paper Record Format

Pros	Cons
Familiarity to users	Content may be unreadable
Portability	Format inelastic
No "downtime"	Access, availability, and retrieval
Flexibility in recording data	No linkages (hot-links) and integration

described by pioneers like Warner Slack and Lawrence Weed.

▪ Risk-reward ratios will need to decrease prior to the widespread adoption of EHRs into the provision of daily medical care.

▪ EHRs are primarily intended to automate the patient record, but potential benefits resulting from an automated record are enormous.

A committee convened by the IOM characterized several key aspects characterizing an ideal EHR. The first is that the EHR should provide an integrated view of patient data, bringing together the many elements of the current paper (and other media) medical record. The record should represent a longitudinal collection of information for and about patients. The EHR should provide ready access to the large and changing body of knowledge pertaining both to the patient's condition and the rules and regulations associated with reimbursement in the time of managed care. It has become clear that both clinician *order* and *data* entry are necessary to take advantage the potential efficiencies of the EHR as well as to ensure that the information in the record is an accurate rendition of the clinician's actions and thoughts.

Communications tools, such as electronic mail and messaging will enhance communications among providers using the EHR in diverse patient care settings and separated by geographic barriers.

Clinical decision support tools providing current knowledge about diseases, treatments, drug interactions, and risk profiles should be integrated into the EHR.

When properly woven into the other components of patient care, decision support tools represent a huge asset in the delivery of safe, cost-effective, evidence-based medicine to patients.

In addition to the processes surrounding the care of an individual patient, the EHR may provide immediate access to population level information for administrative and research applications.

Background

The concept of an EHR has been around for several decades dating back to efforts by pioneers such as Lawrence Weed and Warner Slack in the 1960s (Fig. 9-3). More recently, the IOM issued a report in 1991 (The Computer-Based Patient Record: An Essential Technology for Health Care) calling for the elimination of paper-based records within 10 years. Nevertheless, 2001 has come and gone and there has been little progress toward the goal put forth by the IOM.

There are some settings in which EHRs have been successfully implemented, such as the Veteran's Health Administration, the New England Healthcare Electronic Data Interchange, the Indiana Network

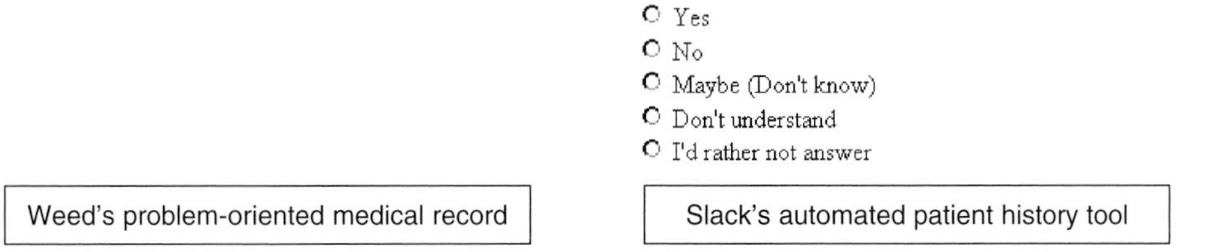

Be Well! Tanger Center Evaluation
Medical History

Problem oriented medical record

#	Problem	Date of onset	Date resolved
1	Cellulitis	01/27/98	02/15/97
2	MI	09/30/01	10/17/01
3	HTN	09/15/01	ongoing

Has anyone in your family (grandparents, uncles, aunts, mother,

father, sisters or brothers) had high blood pressure?

○ Yes
○ No
○ Maybe (Don't know)
○ Don't understand
○ I'd rather not answer

Weed's problem-oriented medical record	Slack's automated patient history tool

Figure 9-3
Early efforts at computerization of medical information date back to the 1960s and 1970s.

for Patient Care, and others. These examples of successful EHR implementations are the exception. In most hospitals, orders, notes, and reports are maintained and reported on paper. Many hospitals lack the capacity to deliver laboratory results to a hospital floor in an automated fashion. Very few small practice environments have undergone any degree of computerization.

The barriers to computerization are formidable. The technical obstacles are relatively obvious. In addition, there are organizational, financial, technological, and policy obstacles. The adoption of an EHR implies a fundamental reorganization of the way medicine is practiced at the point of contact. The clinician must migrate from handwritten notes and orders to procedures involving hands-on contact with a computer.

Many older physicians have had little occasion to use a computer and are therefore likely to be slowed in their performance of formerly routine tasks. This is a major barrier at a time when demands for efficiency are increasing substantially. The costs necessary for hardware, training, and maintenance of an EHR are likely to be substantial and return on investment will be delayed by some period of time. The scope of an EHR implementation in a given environment may vary depending on the vendor and the setting: some EHR implementations will include all patient data, whereas others will be more limited in scope.

The relative inertia in the development of EHRs and their integration into routine healthcare can almost certainly be attributed the high risk versus reward ratio for early adopters. However, the incentives are likely to change in the very near future. Governmental and private stakeholders have begun to develop a combination of grant-based incentives, quality incentive programs, bonuses and low cost capital to encourage the use of certain components of an EHR, such as computerized order entry (CPOE) or quality reporting. A more draconian approach would be to require providers to use EHR systems as a condition of participation in certain insurance plans, such as Medicare.

An essential prerequisite to the general adoption of EHRs is the development of a functional model describing a common set of requirements for the expected capabilities of various subcomponents, such as the ambulatory record. These specifications can be used by vendors to design and by providers to compare products providing a common set of functions.

Tasks of an EHR

Key Points

- The patient's EHR will consist of contributions from site-specific (e.g., office visit, OR record) EHRs as well as data generated by interactions with ancillary services.

- Standardized coding terminology is critical to the viability of EHRs.

The primary task of an EHR is automation of the medical record; however, there are an almost infinite number of functions that can be performed once the paperless medical record becomes prevalent. Principal outcomes described by the aforementioned IOM report include the enhancement of patient care delivery, the management of patient care, efficiency of support processes (i.e., laboratory, radiology, house-keeping, transport, and so on), and the administrative (i.e., billing and reimbursement) requirements that pay for health care.

Examples of secondary benefits that have been described are the use of the EHR as a vehicle for education, regulation (e.g., credentialing of care providers), research (e.g., using electronically accessible patient data), public health and homeland security (with the ability to survey medical records electronically for the emergence of unusual epidemiologic trends), and policy support.

The central EHR will be constructed and continuously updated from the contributions of subcomponent EHRs (Fig. 9-4). Potential contributors include many provider groups, such as hospitals, clinics, nursing homes, as well as records maintained by the individual patient, called a personal health record.

An outpatient EHR may very well come from one vendor, while the inpatient counterpart comes from

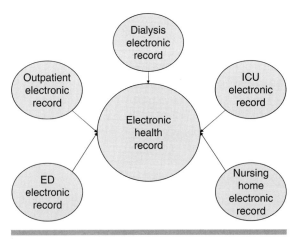

Figure 9-4
An electronic health record can consist of information from component records.

- Decision support (described in Chap. 11)
- Enhanced interprovider communication
- Educational tools for patients and providers
- Administrative support
- Enhanced reporting systems

The core functions expected of EHRs fall into eight general categories. The first and most obvious of these is the management of patient health information and data. This includes medical history, diagnoses, allergies, patient demographics, and test results. Successful EHRs will aggregate and present this complicated body of knowledge in an accessible and readily navigated format (Fig. 9-5). It will most likely evolve in time from something analogous to today's medical chart to something very different as clinicians become familiar with the benefits of computer-based interfaces and willing to use tools like hyperlinked documents.

A second category of EHR functions is the presentation of results acquired from patient testing. Computerization increases the speed and efficiency of results reported by eliminating the delays inherent in manual printing and transmission of data. In many cases, the testing process itself has become partially or fully automated. For example, robotic blood sample analysis dramatically enhances laboratory throughput and shorten time from sample acquisition to results reporting (Fig. 9-6).

A third function of EHRs is CPOE. The traditional ordering paradigm has been the handwritten order. The inefficiencies in this approach are self-evident. The physician writes what is often an illegible order on an order sheet and "flags" the chart to indicate an active order. The order may then sit for some period of time before it is "taken off the chart" by a clerical person. The clerical person then transcribes the order onto a second piece of paper, which is then hand carried to the site that has responsibility for the performance of the procedure of interest, i.e., ECG (Fig. 9-7).

While it represents a significant change in the workflow of a clinician, the success of CPOEs depends to a large extent on the fact that the physician must enter the order into a computer. Many of the potential benefits of CPOEs are realized during the transaction between the clinician

another. The two will need to be integrated to create a coherent EHR, and it is clearly preferable that the same constructs and capabilities extend across the two. This requires uniformity of terminology: it would be unworkable, for example, to use the term "unstable angina" in one part of the record and acute coronary syndrome in another when both refer to the same event. This has led to industry-wide efforts to designate a standard coding terminology such as the Systematized Nomenclature of Medicine (SNOMED). In terms of EHR constructs, it would be preferable to implement hyperlinking as a standard throughout the EHR rather than in one part and not another. Ideally, the same information (such as lab results or an operative note) should not be duplicated in two places, so the EHR engine should consolidate information and eliminate redundancy.

Core EHR Functions

Key Points

- The IOM has described eight core functions of an EHR:
    - *Management* of patient information and data
    - Efficient *presentation* of patient data
    - CPOE (described in Chap. 10)

File No. 1	Name: **JOHN A CITIZEN**		Page No. 1

Date of Birth: 01/01/1941   Address: 22 SUCCESS AVENUE
                                                        DEMOCITY CA 91210

Page Created on: 06/23/01

This scrollable window is for writing case notes.

Medical Condition(s):

This scrollable window is for recording medical condition(s).

Regular Medication(s):

This scrollable window is for recording regular medication(s)

Add New Page |< < View Pages > >|

Monitor: Immunization:

	Wt	BP	BSL	HBA1C	Chol	LDL
03/12/03	120	140/80	7.0	6.5	5.5	3.2
12/09/02	130	150/90	8.0	7.5	7.0	4.0
09/06/02	150	160/100	9.0	8.5	8.5	4.5

12/09/02	ADT
03/11/99	Hep B 3
10/06/99	Hep B 2
09/05/99	Hep B 1

Allergies | Alerts

This scrollable window is for recording allergies and medical alerts...

Scanned Documents:

	Date	Description	Source	
	03/05/03	Full Blood Count	Bethesda Pathology Service	
✎	03/03/03	Xray Chest	Bethesda Radiology Clinic	

Ad Hoc Medication(s):

This scrollable window is for recording ad hoc medication(s).

Figure 9-5
EHRs are usually designed to present comprehensive information to the clinician.

and the computer. What were once illegible orders are now necessarily legible. The potential for lost orders is reduced because there are fewer links in the chain and there is an audit trail. The creation of one order can trigger the implementation of others. Medication orders can be automatically scrutinized for correct dosage, timing, potential drug interactions, allergy conflicts, and relevant laboratory results displayed. Additional benefits include the reduction of costs for forms, clerical personnel, and redundant

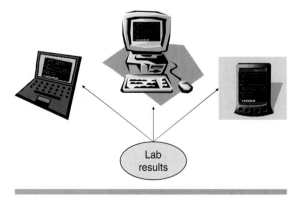

Figure 9-6
Patient results can be "pushed" to the clinician on a variety of devices.

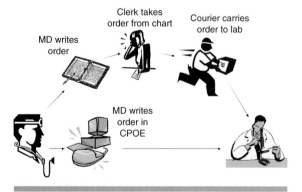

Figure 9-7
The traditional order management approach is much less efficient than the use of a CPOE.

test ordering. Finally, CPOEs provide a logical entry point for automated data entry in the provision of patient care. CPOE implementations will be described more fully in Chap. 10.

A fourth key benefit of EHRs is decision support, where automatically generated reminders and prompts are used to inform the behavior of clinicians (Fig. 9-8). Decision support tools have been used in prevention, drug prescription, diagnosis, disease management. Adherence to preventative practices in areas such as vaccinations, screening, and cardiovascular risk reduction has been improved when decision support tools have been integrated into patient care. More recently, machine learning techniques, such as neural networks, have been used to detect myocardial infarctions, breast cancer, cervical cancer, and nosocomial disease outbreaks. Decision support will be described more fully in Chap. 11.

EHRs can be equipped with communication tools specifically tailored to facilitate communication among the members of the health care team. Email and messaging are typical vehicles for the exchange of patient-related information that can be used to streamline the care of patients who receive care in multiple settings and from multiple providers. These tools can be used for communication among providers from the pharmacy, laboratory, radiology, and clinicians (Fig. 9-9).

Patient support tools for patient education can be integrated into EHRs to teach patients about

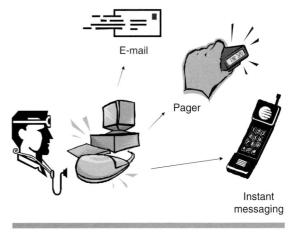

Figure 9-9
Many EHRs provide communication tools that facilitate communication among clinicians.

specific diseases and to facilitate self-testing. These tools can also be used to generate information about new diagnoses and reminders about appointments (Fig. 9-10).

Many administrative processes can be built into EHRs including scheduling systems (Fig. 9-11), billing management, and insurance validation. Automated identification of patients eligible for clinical trials can be done using automated tools.

Finally, internal and external reporting requirements have become increasingly onerous and complicated. Federal, state, and organizational demands for

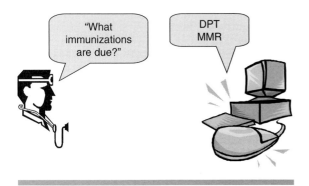

Figure 9-8
Decision support tools can assist the clinician in adherence to routine medical care.

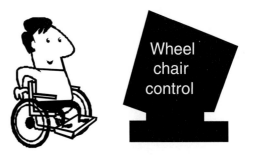

Figure 9-10
Patient education tools can be integrated into EHRs permitting the clinician to provide supplementary material on specific topics.

information place a huge demand on hospitals that can be simplified using reporting systems built into EHRs. Additionally, internal quality improvement programs can use data from EHRs in the analysis and restructuring of care processes (Fig. 9-12).

Criteria for the Successful EHR

The IOM identified five criteria by which EHR functionalities should eventually be judged. The first is their ability to improve patient safety, given growing data that many patients die or are harmed by medical errors, which are much easier to identify and avert with the use of an EHR.

Secondly, it is also increasingly clear that there are wide variations in the way medical care is provided across the United States, and the concept of evidence-based guidelines is a relatively new one. Successful EHRs will act as a vehicle to promulgate and monitor adherence to evidence-based medicine.

Thirdly, medical care is incredibly inefficient relative to other industries of comparable maturity. EHRs will have to pay for themselves to some extent through the efficiencies they generate in the delivery of patient care. Computerization of medical information and processes is a necessary tool as we attempt to address the increasing expenses of medicine.

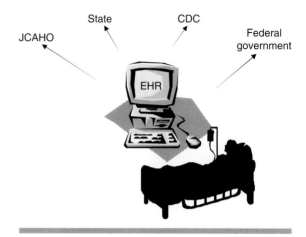

Figure 9-12
EHRs can facilitate the acquisition of data required for various reporting requirements.

Fourth, many patients have multiple, chronic conditions, and the coordination of care for those patients is essential to efficient patient management.

Finally, successful EHR functions will only be implemented when they become viable. For example, certain EHR applications, such as patient self-management tools are not widely offered by vendors as of yet and should not be expected to be an initial part of an EHR implementation. These indicators of success will be realized to various degrees as EHR technology and the several core functionalities mature.

■ Timelines

Key Points

■ EHRs will diffuse into the healthcare sector in three epochs:

- *Near term*: automation of information already in the electronic format, electronic order entry, and prescribing
- *Intermediate term*: penetration of EHRs into nonacute care setting and integration of EHRs from various sources into a unified EHR
- *Far term*: fully integrated EHRs captured longitudinally and with mature decision support as well more universal access

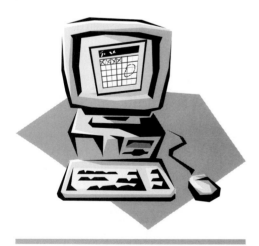

Figure 9-11
Computerized scheduling is one of many administrative tools that can be integrated into and HER.

The IOM committee assigned to evaluate EHRs was asked to project the diffusion of this technology into healthcare systems over the next decade. Their report described three time periods (Fig. 9-13).

In the short term, they believe that providers will focus on the electronic capture of data that is already in an electronic format, such as laboratory and radiology data. Electronic order entry and prescribing will likely be adopted by many providers in the short term, since these systems are already available and reasonably robust. Finally, automated generation of reports for external quality and oversight is a high priority due to the labor-intensive alternative of abstraction from paper records.

In the more intermediate future, the IOM believes that EHR systems will permit the capture of defined sets of health information, incorporate core decision support functions, and permit the electronic exchange of patient care data such as lab results and discharge summaries among diverse care settings (i.e., hospitals, pharmacies, nursing homes, and so on).

In the far term, fully functional, comprehensive EHRs will be developed and adopted in some health systems and/or regions. These EHRs will undoubtedly look different from today's versions and permit longitudinal collection of health information for an individual, immediate and simultaneous access by authorized users within a secure environment, and the integration of tailored decision support tools.

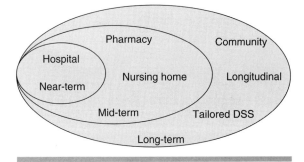

Figure 9-13
The diffusion of EHR technology will proceed in several stages.

Universal Medical Record

Key Points

■ A universal medical record (UMR) should be accessible by an authorized provider at any time from anywhere.

■ The concept of a UMR raises significant and appropriate privacy concerns.

■ A key element to the development of a UMR is correct patient identification through the use of some form of universal patient identifier.

The concept of a UMR deserves specific attention. Discussions about an EHR do not typically address the issues of storage and ownership of the data. Legally, a medical record belongs to the institution in which it is generated or the physician who maintains it, in the case of a private office. The patient has specific access rights, however, which vary from country to country. As the EHR migrates from a location-bound, paper document to an electronic document it will integrate information from many locations and may reside in none of them (Fig. 9-14).

As EHRs proliferate and mature, so will models permitting increased portability of the record or its components. It has always been desirable for providers in one location to have access to data from a medical record generated at another location. A hospital-based clinician may wish to have access to outpatient records from the same health system. Alternatively, clinicians currently caring for a patient may need to have access to the records from a previous hospitalization in a different geographic location and health system. The first scenario will eventually be addressed by the adoption of an integrated EHR for the specific health system. However, both scenarios can be addressed by the development of a UMR that is geographically independent and controlled by the patient.

There are many possible models for a UMR. Given the rapid evolution of memory technologies, it is possible to imagine the development of totally portable devices on which a patient's entire record is stored. The patient could then be responsible for the storage and management of the record and

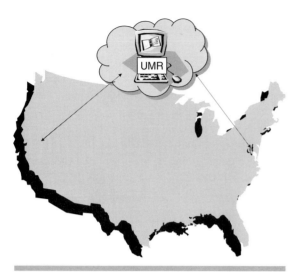

Figure 9-14
The universal medical record can reside almost anywhere but should also be accessible by authorized parties from anywhere at any time.

carry it from visit to visit. The problems with this model are obvious, such as what happens if the record is lost, stolen, or destroyed. Similarly, what happens if the patient develops a life-threatening medical condition and the medical record is not immediately available? There are also potential problems with standardization of compatible interface hardware at potential encounter-points between the patient and the medical system. Finally, the need to have the card present at the time of data review makes third party consultation (i.e., between primary and consulting physician) problematic.

A more practical arrangement is to place the UMR somewhere on the Internet, where it can be accessed when necessary. Several desirable attributes of a UMR have been described. There is a consensus that the information stored in a UMR should adhere to some standard in terms of content and structure, while simultaneously permitting sufficient flexibility that various documentation styles can be accommodated. The UMR clearly must adhere to industry-wide data standards for data names, disease nomenclature, and image formats.

In order to qualify as a UMR, the "document" must be able to be stored anywhere and retrievable from anywhere, implying that it must be accessible over a common network used by healthcare networks and providers. In order to ensure data security and integrity, common mechanisms must be in place at all terminals (i.e., data warehouses, hospitals, doctor's offices, and so on) to encode and decode the record after passage over the common network. Since care and documentation will be provided in different languages, the UMR must not be constrained to a single language.

Assuming that the UMR is stored somewhere on the Internet, which is the only network currently meeting the requirements listed above, the record will no longer be "owned" by providers, and ownership and control will rest with the patient. The information contained in the record can be divided into several categories with different degrees of sensitivity. The patient will probably want to provide ready, automatic access to information such as diagnoses and allergies to authenticated providers with a legitimate need for the requested information. Conversely, the patient will probably want to put secure "barriers" around certain information, such as data relating to psychiatric conditions or HIV status. It has become increasingly apparent that any information on the Internet will be subjected to unauthorized access attempts, and the cost-benefit ratio to on-line medical storage must outweigh the potential risks; and the risks here apply to both the patient and the providers whose actions are documented in the record. The patient and provider should therefore agree what aspects of their interaction will be recorded in the on-line UMR.

In the event that a provider requires access to a UMR, access rights and authentication are essential issues. It is possible that a patient could provide a list of authorized, trusted parties who may have access to the record. This approach has flaws however. For example, it is unclear how to prevent malicious access by a hacker masquerading as a trusted party. More importantly, this approach does not provide for access by new but legitimate providers in the event of a health care emergency when the patient is unable to authorize access. An alternative would be to prospectively establish access rules which would require specific patient identifiers, the location from which access is requested, and credentials of the requestor.

Accurate patient identification is challenging and the problem grows with the size of the potential database. The traditional approach in U.S. hospitals has been to use the patient's name, address, and date of birth. However, this approach guarantees retrieval of multiple duplicates in large databases. Master patient indexes are used to store all of the relevant patient medical record numbers in a single database, and are particularly useful when a patient has been cared for at several facilities within an integrated delivery network, where each facility may use a distinct identification scheme. Some countries, such as the United Kingdom, have developed a national patient index with a single health identifier for each patient in the system.

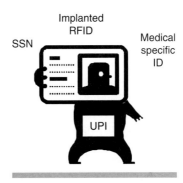

Figure 9-15
The development of a UMR will necessitate the creation of a universal patient identifier (UPI) which could take one of several forms, including existing identifiers (i.e., SSN), the creation of a new one, or the use of new technology like implanted radio-frequency ID tags.

Universal Health Identifier

The Health Insurance Portability and Accountability Act (HIPAA) legislation identified the need for a national universal patient identifier (UPI) as a way of preventing misidentification errors and decreasing the fragmentation of medical information. Alternatives in the United States include the use of existing uniquely identifying attributes, such as the social security number (SSN), or the creation of new ones. The SSN is attractive because the infrastructure to create and use it is already in existence. Some of the downsides, however, include the fact that it can be used to link disparate and broad-ranging databases about an individual including nonmedical data, increasing the potential for malicious misuse. Additionally, the SSN does not include a self-check digit (which insures its integrity) and the mechanisms to create a new SSN at birth and eliminate numbers at death are not currently in existence. Finally, there are not enough SSNs for the foreseeable future (Fig. 9-15).

Another question relating to the UMR relates to its content. An on-line, UMR providing for access by previously unknown providers will by necessity be more vulnerable than a electronic

record residing within the confines of a health system intranet, where all providers are known to the system. A patient may therefore choose to limit the granularity (degree of detail) of the record or constrain the contents (i.e., not include psychiatric data).

Standards and the UMR

In order to be universally understood, the UMR will need to adhere to standards. These standards will have to apply to several aspects of the construction and communication of the UMR. The creation of standards will allow different vendors to create software components for the UMR. It is likely that the vendors who sell software for the storage of the UMR are not the same as those who create client software to access and display the record. Standards will ensure that the same data element is handled in the same way regardless of the vendor. Different standards will need to be adopted for communications (i.e., HTTP), display (i.e., HTML), data categorization (i.e., HL7), and medical terminology (i.e., ICD, CPT, UMLS, SnoMed, and so on).

◼ Conclusion

The electronic medical record is inevitable and its form will change with the evolution of computing tools. Hardware is becoming faster and more portable. Networking speed and security are improving. New tools have emerged for communication, like instant messaging and voice over Internet. Video conferencing and telemedicine applications are being integrated into care delivery. The EHR and UMR will need to evolve from the current paper record format to an electronic counterpart with some general evolutionary pressures. Successful electronic record formats will meet the needs of the patient, the provider, and the public. The patient will want to have a secure record with which he can interact and participate in his own health care management. The provider will want to have ready access to a patient's data and decision support tools to assist in the provision of care. Finally the public will want data pertaining to general healthcare trends as well as the ability to recognize threats to the community from bioterrorism or emerging diseases using tools built into the national health information infrastructure.

◼ Suggested Readings

Amatayakul MK. *Electronic Health Records: A Practical Guide for Professionals and Organizations*. American Health Information Management Association, 2004.

Walker JM, Bieber EJ, Richards F. *Implementing an Electronic Health Record System*. Springer, 2004.

Carter JH. *Electronic Medical Records: A Guide for Clinicians and Administrators*. American College of Physicians, 2001.

CPOE

Introduction

Key Points

- CPOEs are an essential element to the computerization of medical care.
- CPOEs are widely supported as an approach to the standardization of care, to improve the efficiency of care, and to reduce errors in care delivery.

Computerized provider order entry (CPOE) systems are believed to be critical to reducing the number of errors in medical care. Prescribing errors are the most common source of adverse drug events, which have been estimated to injure or kill more than 770,000 patients in hospitals annually. CPOEs with or without decision support tools are widely viewed as being integral to reduction in prescribing errors and formulary control. Some of the diverse advocate groups include researchers, clinicians, hospital administrators, pharmacists, business groups, governmental representatives, health care agencies, the Institute of Medicine, and the lay public (Fig. 10-1).

CPOEs are expected to have various beneficial effects in the delivery of health care including an increase in the efficiency of care, job satisfaction, and error reduction. The improvement in efficiency is obviously desirable given new resident working-hour limitations and nursing shortages.

History

Key Points

- Early CPOEs were "home-grown" at academic institutions.

- There are prominent examples of successes and failures in early CPOEs.
- It is clear that predictors of success include well-designed software, clinician input, and institutional buy-in are critical.

The early development of CPOEs occurred at institutions that developed their own software such as Brigham and Women's Hospital (BWH) in Boston, Latter Day Saints Hospital in Salt Lake City, and Regenstrief Institute for Health Care in Indianapolis. The rights to all three of these systems have been purchased by companies and they are being commercialized. These early adopters were academic medical centers with a captive workforce consisting of residents and faculty physicians, and each has demonstrated success in some fashion.

There are also several cautionary tales of CPOEs that were implemented and failed at some point, the most well publicized being the system at Cedars-Sinai Medical Center which was derailed after a staff revolt. Cedars-Sinai was a pioneer in computerized clinician support systems and developed a $34 million CPOE that was turned off after 3 months of operation. Critics pointed out that the system had several fatal flaws, many of which violate Octo Barnett's rules of good medical system programming outlined in Chap. 8.

The system was apparently developed with little input from physicians, it ran slowly, training was inadequate, and deployment was done with an all-at-once approach. One interesting complaint was the fact that the decision support system was unwieldy, and once an alert was triggered, the clinician became enmeshed in a series of secondary questions generated by the original alert and was unable to proceed with the task originally undertaken.

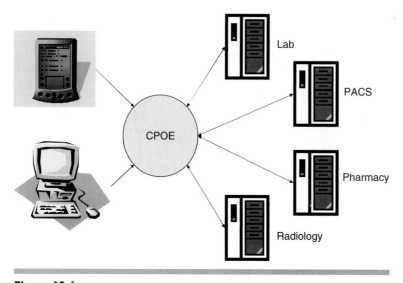

Figure 10-1
A CPOE typically interacts with a variety of other hospital computer systems.

While this is the most well-known example of a failed implementation of medical software statistics suggest that up to 30% of new EHRs fail to some extent.

The Regenstrief Institute in Indiana began work on a computerized medical records system in 1972, initially focusing on the capture and display of patient data. The development efforts moved on to decision support and order entry, primarily driven by the fact that order entry was well understood and structured, and therefore more susceptible to the development of computerized tools. Regenstrief also recognized that structured orders are likely to result in restructured and standardized practice patterns.

Over time, the Regenstrief development team identified successful approaches for new component development—which might be new interfaces, rules, or order sets. They used rapid prototyping with active clinician involvement. They also had consistent, strong executive level support within the institution, and a focus on the improvement of care processes, technical excellence, and responsiveness to users' needs.

BWH was another early adopter that developed a customized order entry system in the mid-1990s.

The initial costs for development were estimated at $1.5M, but the system is believed to save $5–10M per year. It incorporates a decision support system and has several modes for order entry, including "assisted mode" (prompts for required fields), "quick mode" (allows free text), and templated order sets.

The BWH system was designed to require minimal training and was extensively studied after implementation. Some of the early findings were the avoidance of adverse drug events through an allergy warning system, savings from appropriate drug prescriptions, and process standardization (Fig. 10-2).

There are some recent data suggesting that CPOEs may have unexpected effects relating to design or implementation issues. In a 2005 *JAMA* study, researchers at the University of Pennsylvania identified information errors and human-machine interface errors in an early CPOE system. Among the former, they found issues relating to default drug-dosing, failure to discontinue medications, failure to renew medications, duplicate drug orders, and allergy warnings that were ignored because they were presented after the drug was ordered (Fig. 10-3).

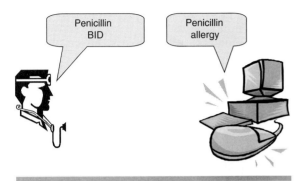

Figure 10-2
The CPOE can be configured to provide decision support messages such as allergy alerts.

Human factor issues (such as the size of screen fonts) caused incorrect patient selection, and/or medication selection (Fig. 10-4). Additional design flaws resulted in log/off failures, dysfunctional system outage processes, and inflexible ordering

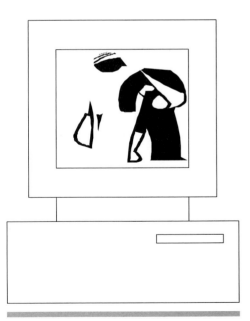

Figure 10-3
Some research has shown that poorly designed CPOE interfaces can provide an incomplete or incoherent view of the patient.

screens. Some of these issues related to the fact that the studied CPOE was an older, nonwindowed system and data were presented inefficiently, often spanning several screens (such as a patient medication list). Nevertheless, it is clear a poorly designed CPOE can impede the performance of the clinician, and, even worse, lead the clinician into patient care errors.

■ Definition

Key Points

■ The term CPOE encompasses systems with a range of capabilities, including simple order entry to combinations of results reporting, order entry, and decision support (further described in Chap. 11).

■ CPOEs can speed the delivery of orders, enhance legibility and accuracy, and reduce duplicate or inappropriate orders.

■ Published data on the prevalence on medical errors has increased the interest of the government, industry, and insurers in widespread adoption of CPOEs.

The term CPOE is used generically to refer to a variety of different computer-based ordering systems designed to automate the ordering process. They may include the ability to order drugs, pathology tests, radiology tests in addition to providing results reporting.

The expected benefits of such a system include the output of standardized, complete, legible orders that are consistent with the hospital's formulary and automatically sent to the pharmacy. The orders reach the pharmacy more rapidly than paper-based orders do, are presumably less subject to confusion due to similar sounding drugs, are more likely to correctly identify the prescribing physician, can be linked to adverse drug event reporting systems, and reduce over-prescription (and under-prescription) (Fig. 10-5).

CPOEs are almost invariably associated with a decision support system, or DSS (Chap. 11), which can be as simple as a system that suggests default values for drug doses, routes, and frequencies or a much more sophisticated program used to implement practice guidelines. Advanced DSSs can

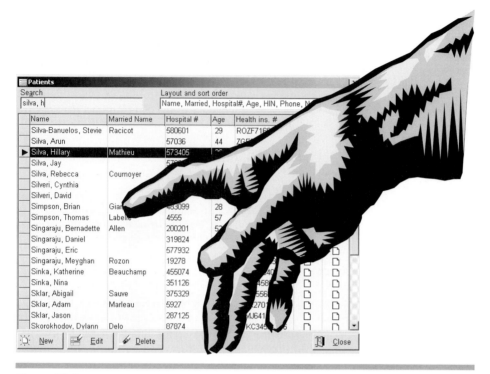

Figure 10-4
Human factor issues, such as a large screen pointer combined with small fonts can cause incorrect patient selection and resulting order errors.

check for patient drug allergies (based on profile information), compare drug and laboratory values, and evaluate the potential for drug-drug interactions. Additionally, DSSs can provide recommendations about corollary order sets, such as glucose

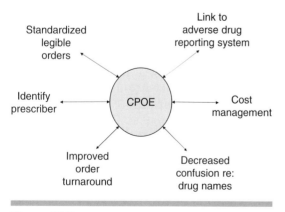

Figure 10-5
There are a variety of benefits to the use of a CPOE.

checks with insulin therapy, and suggest drug guidelines to the clinician at the time the drug is ordered. Suggestions might include drug alternatives, dosage alterations, and so on. Additional potential benefits include improved communication among caregivers, improved quality of care, and reduced cost of the delivery of care.

The aforementioned early adopters had good success with their home-grown systems, some of which have been licensed by commercial software providers. However, it is clear that there are potential pitfalls associated with the adoption of CPOEs as well, as at the Cedars-Sinai deployment and as shown by the data from the first generation CPOE studied at Penn.

Whatever the data, CPOEs have come into the spotlight following the Institute of Medicine's 1999 report To Err is Human: Building a Safer Health System, in which 44,000–98,000 deaths per year were attributed to medical errors. CPOEs were identified as one potential solution to the problem.

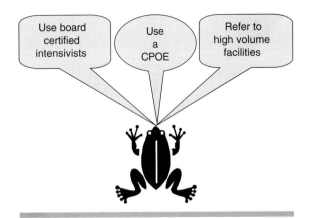

Figure 10-6
The Leapfrog group, representing large employers, created three initial standards to improve patient care.

Subsequently, the Leapfrog Group (which represents a large consortium of health care buyers) selected CPOEs as a safety standard (Fig. 10-6). The government is now studying incentives for hospitals that implement CPOEs. The question is no longer whether or not to purchase a CPOE, it is which one and how to get it right.

Implementation

Key Points

- The deployment of a new CPOE can be fraught with problems.
- The American Medical Informatics Association developed a list of nine key considerations that should be evaluated prior to deployment of a CPOE:
    - What is the institutional motivation?
    - Is the correct leadership in place to sustain a CPOE?
    - Is the CPOE adequately funded?
    - How will the proposed CPOE impact on workflow in affected areas?
    - What is the cost-benefit ratio for the various user groups?
    - What is the rollout plan and is it staged?
    - Are the technical aspects (i.e., response time, new user authorization) acceptable?
    - What is the training plan?
    - Is the system readily susceptible to continuous change and improvement?

According to those who have succeeded, the key to successful deployment of a CPOE is to recognize that it is more than the purchase of a piece of software; rather it represents a fundamental redesign of patient care delivery processes. There are both technical and organizational aspects to the deployment of a system. A recent consensus panel developed a list of nine issues that CPOE experts believe must be considered before implementation of such a system in a health system.

The first consideration is a firm understanding of the motivation behind the implementation of a CPOE. This will influence where funding derives from, internal political and clinical leadership. Potential external drivers include requirements from regional or national authorities, such as Leapfrog, Medicare, or the JCAHO. Alternatively, competitors in the region might advertise their use of a CPOE, creating pressure for adoption of a CPOE locally. Internal pressure could come from administrative or clinical leaders and their objectives should be clear, i.e., are they looking for improved efficiency.

The second consideration relates to the internal leadership required to sustain support over the extended period of time needed to evaluate, purchase, and deploy a CPOE. Leadership is necessary at the executive level, champion level, project management level, and clinical level. Exe-cutive leaders must commit firmly and visibly to the implementation of a CPOE and communicate a vision of the goals of the CPOE as they integrate with those of the organization as a whole. The articulation of this vision might include the deficiencies in the current approach (i.e., paper) and the anticipated benefits of the CPOE in remediating those deficiencies. It is critical to identify a CPOE project leader with the ability to assess the ongoing success of the project, educate and foster teamwork. The key players must be realistic about what is involved in the deployment of a CPOE: the degree of change involved, the preexisting organizational success with change, and the resources necessary to effect change.

Internal clinical champions must be identified and engaged. These are respected individuals whose support for the CPOE is likely to increase the chances of success. It is essential to determine whether the organization has the money, technical infrastructure, project management skills, and staff readiness to adopt a CPOE. Where deficient, the organization should hire or consult individuals who can assist during deployment. Finally, it is critical to select a vendor with a track record of success who will engage as a full partner throughout the deployment of the CPOE.

The third consideration is the costs of the CPOE. The costs include both software and hardware, where necessary, as well as hidden costs relating to training and productivity losses during installation. An underfunded rollout will be chaotic at best and is likely to fail because personnel are untrained or resistant when training impacts on their personal time.

The fourth consideration is critical and pertains to the way the CPOE integrates into the systems workflow and health care delivery. Without careful, site-by-site evaluation of the way in which the CPOE will affect the workflow processes of the clinicians (Fig. 10-7) and clerical personnel, the system is vulnerable to failure. A system-wide change management strategy can facilitate the integration of this major alteration in care into the delivery of health care. The technical aspects of integration have to do with the way in which the CPOE will interact with existing HIS applications such as the laboratory and pharmacy systems. Finally, it is essential to clarify downtime procedures that are appropriate to each site.

The fifth consideration relates to the cost-benefit ratio of the CPOE for each user. Specifically, the use of the CPOE might cost additional transaction time (i.e., to log onto the system), but have benefits that outweigh that cost (i.e., by the ability to use an order set rather than create several individual orders). Decision support tools are likely to be of benefit, for example, by freeing the clinician from having to look up a new drug prior to prescribing it. It is critical that the clinicians using the system understand the benefits of decision support, that the DSS paradigms are consistent (i.e., consistent

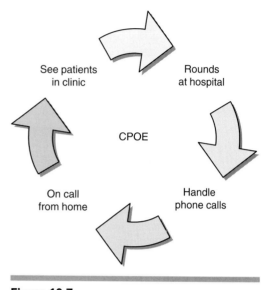

Figure 10-7
In order to be accepted, a CPOE must be integrated into and facilitate the workflow of clinician.

methods for the identification of allergies, drug-drug interactions, expensive tests, duplicate meds, and so on) and that order sets are reviewed and maintained. These cost-benefit trade-offs should be clarified to the user pool prior to go-live, because the "costs" are likely to be highest during the initial period when unfamiliarity results in transient inefficiencies that may be extremely frustrating to new users.

The sixth consideration is the approach to project management and staged implementation (Fig. 10-8). The experts on the consensus panel were extremely attentive to the people involved in implementation, the intermediary goals of the staged deployment, the measurement of the success of each step, and the preparation of the personnel for deployment. They can see that it is essential to establish a culture for ongoing system evaluation and improvement.

The seventh consideration relates to technical details. Some critical examples include the plan for the authorization of new users, the development of interfaces with other and new systems, whether there is a need for remote access, and the details of

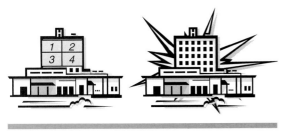

Figure 10-8
There are two general approaches to deployment of a CPOE-staged implementations and all-at-once ("big bang") rollouts.

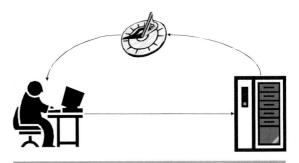

Figure 10-9
CPOEs, and any other software for that matter, should have a rapid response time to be accepted in a busy clinical environment.

the user interface. Another key issue is finding the right balance between using the off-the-shelf software and customizing the system. There are trade-offs to both approaches. Customization is expensive and may degrade system performance, while standard software may not be suitable for the hospital system. Additionally, it is important to understand the plan for replacing a legacy system and the degree to which the new application can interface with existing or planned systems. It is also important to know what kind of performance to expect from an application in the local environment, i.e., what kind of response time and user interface performance. Response times should be less than 1 s (Fig. 10-9). The software interface should be very consistent across modules, and there should be an adequate number of workstations to permit easy access to clinicians. Some hospitals have chosen to provide mobile workstations for certain user groups and applications.

The eighth consideration relates to training and support. New systems are most vulnerable during the initial implementation period when the new user group is unfamiliar with the software. Regardless of the level of pre-go-live training, the essential period of support immediately follows go-live, and experts recommend 24-hour support for several days following the deployment of a new, mission-critical piece of software (like a CPOE) in a hospital setting. Specific consideration should be given to support for clinical and technical personnel, online help, and mentoring (sometimes called super-users). Formal training is less useful than

personal coaching during the rollout period, and trusted clinicians (super-users) are better coaches than applications specialists in many cases. New staff should receive CPOE training as part of their orientation.

The final consensus consideration pertains to continuous improvement following go-live. Good systems continue to evolve after installation and have plans for continuous evaluation, formal feedback, and reconsideration of initial design decisions (Fig. 10-10).

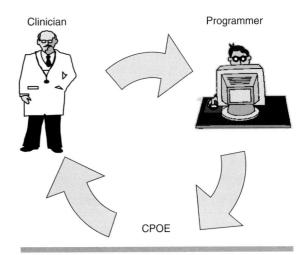

Figure 10-10
Successful medical software is subjected to continuous reevaluation and quality improvement.

The key, underlying message to each of these considerations is the fact that CPOE implementation implies system-wide change, and the institution must therefore participate as a whole. Executive and clinician (nurse, physician) leadership are critical to the process. An implementation that is perceived to be an information system effort will almost inevitably fail.

Conclusion

Some of the themes derived from successful pioneer CPOEs are the following. There were clear ties between the institution's strategic plan and the adoption of the CPOE. The people and process changes inherent in converting to CPOE should be perceived as improvements in patient care rather than the implementation of new technology. Clinician participation and leadership during the process are highly correlated with smooth and successful implementation. Finally, the perception that the vendor and information services are partners in the installation and flexible about design changes and customization are important.

Suggested Readings

Carlton F, Hotchkiss LS, Sheff RA. *Lessons Learned: A Guide to Evaluating and Implementing CPOE*. Hcpro, 2004. http://www.ahrq.gov/clinic/ptsafety/chap6.htm.

11 Decision Support Systems

Introduction

Key Points

- Medical knowledge has traditionally been memorized and the clinician is expected to keep that knowledge current.
- New medical knowledge and "best practices" are developing at a rapid pace.
- Decision support tools can be used to provide medical information and "best practice standards" at the point of care.

Traditional medical training requires the memorization of vast bodies of information and regurgitation or application more or less on demand. The best medical students are often those with the most prodigious memories: "roundsmanship" is prized. However, medical information has become so complicated and changes so rapidly that it is impossible to stay current. Additionally, the concept of "best-practice" is increasingly replacing that of "the way I do it," and the definition of best practice is, in and of itself, difficult to keep up with. Many estimate that much of the information that a clinician graduates from school with is obsolete within a decade.

Computerized decision support (as contrasted with decision making) is the obvious answer. Decision support tools can be kept current by people or technologies dedicated to that task, and clinicians can tap in on that current information on demand, rather than needing to maintain their own, memory-based version of current medical knowledge (Fig.11-1).

History

Key Points

- Early decision support tools were developed at several places including the University of Pittsburgh and Stanford.
- These systems were designed to codify bodies of medical information and act as consultants.

The first systems developed to assist in medical decision making date back to the early days of artificial intelligence in the 1970s and 80s, because the practice of medicine was recognized early on to be a logical application for smart technology.

Two systems designed to assist medical decision making deserve mention. The first was developed at the University of Pittsburgh, by Dr. Jack Myers and a computer engineer named Harry Pople, as well as Dr. Randall Miller and called INTERNIST-1. This system was developed in 1974 and designed to address diagnostic dilemmas in the fields of internal medicine and neurology. It used what was been characterized as the "hypotheco-deductive" approach, wherein observations about a patient, such as signs and symptoms, were used to deduce a set of compatible diseases. By prioritizing the possibilities and asking additional questions, the system narrowed the possibility list to a few possibilities or a single best choice. When compared to experts using cases from the *New England Journal*, the system performed competently, but it was never widely integrated into medical practice.

Another medical decision support system (DSS), MYCIN, was designed by Dr. Edward Shortliffe

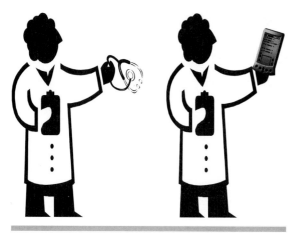

Figure 11-1
The standard medical pocket instrument used to be the stethoscope and is increasingly the PDA.

at Stanford University in the mid-1970s (Fig. 11-2). It functioned as an infectious disease specialist and used an underlying set of IF-THEN rule pairs with weighting factors. The system was designed to be used by internists, and has been characterized as a

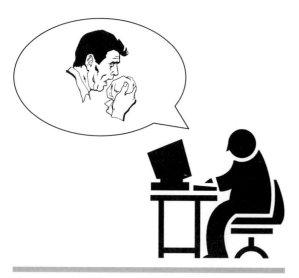

Figure 11-2
MYCIN is an expert system designed at Stanford to reproduce the thinking of an infectious disease consultant.

goal-directed AI system, in which the rule set was searched for relevant rules which were used to drive the system toward a solution.

The INTERNIST-1 system was eventually commercialized as quick medical reference (QMR) and was maintained until recently as a product for the personal computer (Fig. 11-3). Another clinically oriented diagnostic DSS was developed at Massachusetts General Hospital in the 1980s and is sold under the name Dxplain. It knows about approximately 2200 diseases and 5000 symptoms (Fig. 11-4). However, despite three decades of work on diagnostic decisions support systems they have not been widely integrated into medical practice.

Many reasons have been put forth for the relative failure of these systems, but the most likely and all encompassing is the relatively slow penetration of computers into medical practice. Newer DSSs with a more targeted scope are being developed and will likely come into widespread use as components of other medical software.

Decision Support Functions

Key Points

- Decision support tools are currently used in four major roles:
    - Administrative support for clinicians
    - Patient care management
    - Order management
    - Support of "best practice" delivery
- The limited data that are available suggest the DSSs improve patient outcomes and the efficiency of care.
- Decision support software is slowly being integrated into computerized provider order entry (CPOEs) and electronic health records (EHRs).
- The logic underpinning a DSS varies depending on the type of support being rendered by the system.

Four major functions of DSSs can be described. The first is an administrative role, wherein DSSs support clinical coding and documentation as well as the management of patient referrals and authorization for procedures. A primary care physician might use an automated decision support tool, for

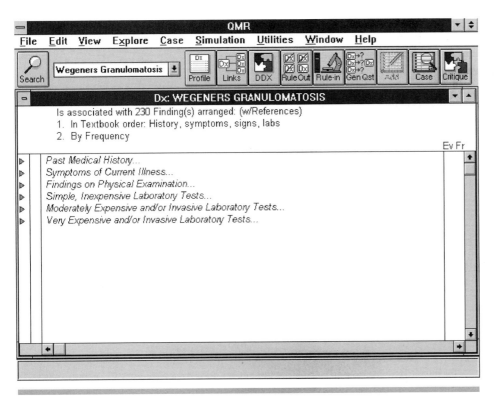

Figure 11-3
Quick medical record is the commercial version of Internist which is an expert system designed to diagnose medical and neurologic diseases.

example, to determine whether a patient is appropriate for referral to a consultant (Fig. 11-5).

The second major category for DSSs is to assist in controlling the complex and varied aspects of medical care, such as automatically scheduling follow-up visits, tracking orders to completion and report-out, automatically generating reminders relative to preventative care (i.e., inoculations), or tracking adherence to research protocols (Fig. 11-6).

A third general category, and perhaps the best recognized is the role of DSS tools in cost control and avoidance by the management of pharmacy, laboratory, and other test ordering or the elimination of duplicate and unnecessary tests (Fig. 11-7).

Finally, DSSs will come into widespread use in the promotion of best-practices (i.e., stress-ulcer prophylaxis), condition-specific guidelines (i.e., asthma),

and population-based management (i.e., blacks with hypertension).

State of the Art

The computerization of the clinical environment has proceeded slowly relative to other industries, as previously noted. The necessary underpinning for widespread adoption of DSSs is the use of the software on which they typically ride, i.e. EHRs and order entry systems. If the DSS is not integrated into the workflow, the clinician is unlikely to engage with it. One expert on the diffusion of decision support technology stated it succinctly: "if a technology is easily assimilated into the existing practice, it will be quickly embraced; if it disrupts everyday activities, the social organization,

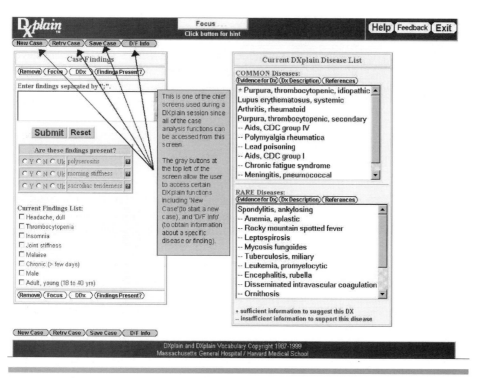

Figure 11-4
DxPlain is a diagnostic expert system designed at Harvard.

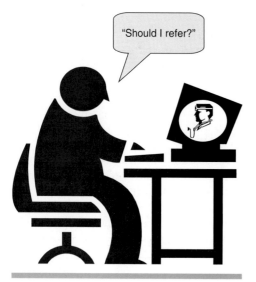

Figure 11-5
Decision support systems can be used to determine when to refer a patient to a consultant.

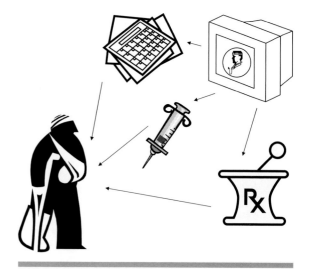

Figure 11-6
Some decision support systems are designed to ensure that patients stay on a pathway.

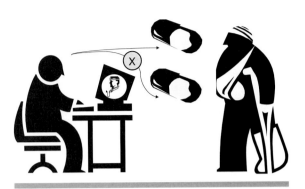

Figure 11-7
Some decision support systems suggest drug alternatives or block duplicate orders.

or status quo, it will not be."[1] This is not to say that DSSs can't act as stand-alone software as did the early diagnostic systems listed above. However, it is the point of contact between the clinician and the computer where DSSs are most effective and most likely to be accepted.

DSSs integrated into EHRs and CPOEs will probably be the first widely deployed products of this description. They may assist with the determination of proper drug dosing, remind clinicians to engage in preventative interventions for their patients, alert clinicians regarding potential adverse events, give feedback on orders by the clinician, prompt for treatments or testing, and/or assist in diagnosing a patient's condition. Successful DSSs will need to save both time and money. The time savings will act as direct incentives to the clinicians, whereas the monetary savings will more likely accrue to the purchaser, be it a physician practice or hospital. Parenthetically, systems that are perceived to act primarily as watchdogs intended to monitor clinician behavior or compliance will almost certainly meet with resistance.

Systems have been developed and integrated into the workflow at several sites, such as the Health Evaluation through Logical Processing (HELP) system at Latter Day Saints Hospital in Salt Lake City, and the WizOrder system at Vanderbilt. The HELP

system integrates DSS into a comprehensive medical record, whereas WizOrder is primarily an order entry system (Fig. 11-8). Both systems were developed in-house over a period of decades and are therefore highly tailored to the local practice environment. For many reasons, many of the initial development of DSSs took place at academic centers. Commercial vendors have begun to enter into the decision support sector, and have licensed or acquired preexisting DSSs or are developing their own.

There are limited data as to the benefit of DSSs, but studies have shown that computerized systems can improve clinician performance and positively affect patient outcomes. These benefits tend to flow from DSS interventions relating to drug dosing and prescribing, diagnostic assistance, reminders about preventative care, and increased adherence to clinical or best-practice protocols. There is also evidence that DSSs can improve the efficiency of care by reducing the amount of time clinicians spend on administrative tasks and the turn-around time between test ordering and performance.

DSSs have also been shown to reduce the costs of medical care. Most of the demonstrated savings result from the increased prescription of less expensive drugs and tests relative to controls, although there is also data relating to the reduction of medication errors and adverse events.

Most of the studies showing cost-benefit from DSSs have been done at institutions where the systems were developed internally and had been through a period of substantial refinement. The alerts were customized and "applied" judiciously. It has become apparent that there is a balance between the absence of alerts and the production of too many. At some point, increases in the number of alerts results in an overall diminishment in compliance, presumably due to attention overload.

Types of Decision Support Systems

Key Points

- DSSs can be categorized as state analysis machines or strategy management systems.
- DSSs have the following characteristics:
  - They use input data
  - They have a knowledge base

[1]Weaver R. *Computers and Medical Knowledge: The Diffusion of Decision Support Technology*. Boulder, CO: Westview Press, 1991.

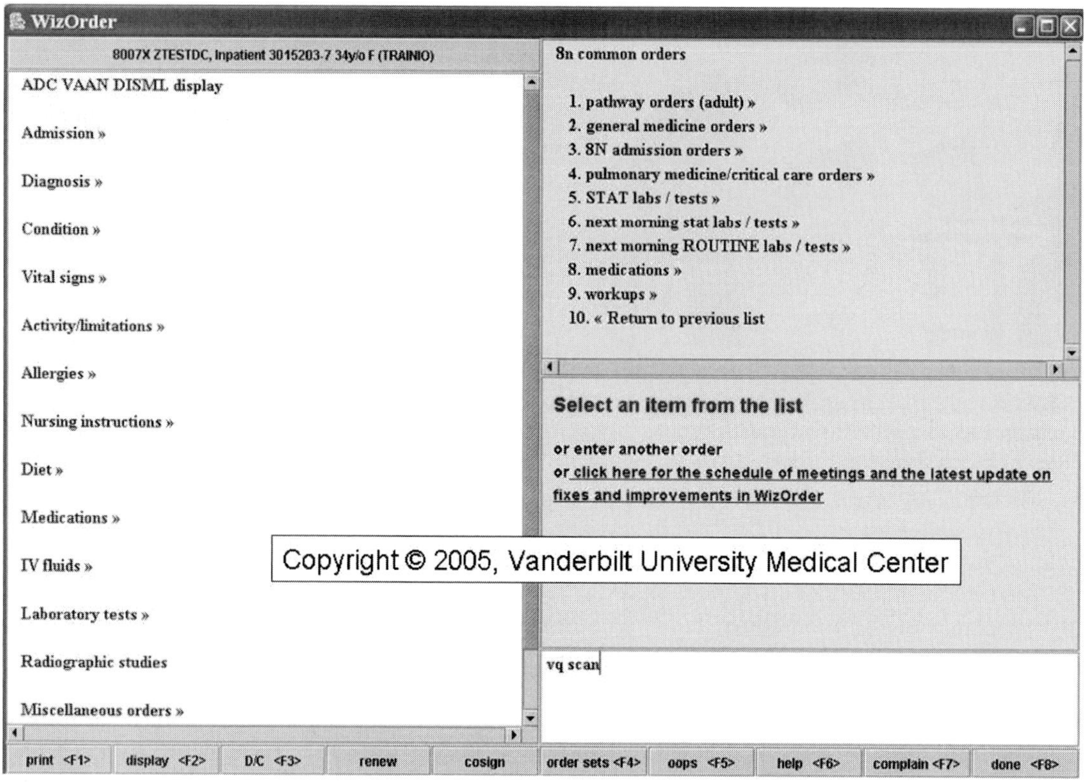

WizOrder

| 8007X ZTESTDC, Inpatient 3015203-7 34y/o F (TRAINIO) | |

ADC VAAN DISML display

Admission »

Diagnosis »

Condition »

Vital signs »

Activity/limitations »

Allergies »

Nursing instructions »

Diet »

Medications »

IV fluids »

Laboratory tests »

Radiographic studies

Miscellaneous orders »

8n common orders

1. pathway orders (adult) »
2. general medicine orders »
3. 8N admission orders »
4. pulmonary medicine/critical care orders »
5. STAT labs / tests »
6. next morning stat labs / tests »
7. next morning ROUTINE labs / tests »
8. medications »
9. workups »
10. « Return to previous list

Select an item from the list

or enter another order
or click here for the schedule of meetings and the latest update on fixes and improvements in WizOrder

Copyright © 2005, Vanderbilt University Medical Center

vq scan

| print <F1> | display <F2> | D/C <F3> | renew | cosign | order sets <F4> | oops <F5> | help <F6> | complain <F7> | done <F8> |

Figure 11-8
This screenshot shows an order screen from Vanderbilt's WizOrder system (courtesy Dr. Randall Miller).

- They have a logical "engine"
- They generate recommendations or interventions

■ DSSs can use a top-down or bottom-up approach to knowledge acquisition

■ Passive systems wait to be asked for input

■ Semiactive systems "speak-up" when they "notice" something

■ Active systems intervene automatically

One logical way of classifying approaches to decision support is to differentiate between those systems that attempt to analyze or predict a patient's present or future state and those that attempt to direct the strategy for care giving. The systems described at the beginning of the chapter (MYCIN and INTERNIST-1) are *state analysis machines* (Fig. 11-9), whereas systems directing the care of a

patient using guidelines or protocols are *strategy management systems* (Fig. 11-10). Many systems make use of both approaches.

Regardless of type, the DSS must begin with a knowledge base, use some kind of an "engine" and produce or effect recommendations or interventions.

The knowledge may consist of observations (such as automated observations about a patient's vital signs or manually entered observations from a clinician). Alternatively, a system can be primed with academically derived knowledge (as was the INTERNIST-1 system) typically contained in books or medical journals. Either of these knowledge bases can be enhanced with experiential knowledge (as with self-teaching software or experience derived from the practice of medicine) (Fig. 11-11).

The "engine" is the underlying software and analysis methodology. It can generally be thought

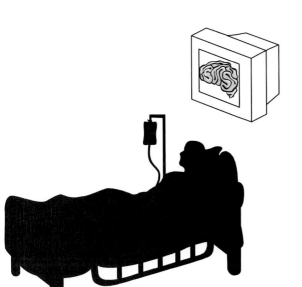

Figure 11-9
A state analysis system can sit in the background monitoring lab or vital sign trends and alerting when appropriate.

of as a black box from the clinician's vantage point, although it is valuable to understand some of the common approaches as well as those that will become increasingly prevalent in the future. Finally, the types of interventions a DSS can make are broadly classifiable into passive, semiactive, and active systems.

Medical decision making requires the use of many different types of knowledge. A clinician may, for example, use anatomic, pathologic, epidemiologic, taxonomic, pharmacologic, and therapeutic information in reaching a diagnosis or decision about treatment. A DSS should be capable of using these same datasets. The cognitive component of a DSS can use empirical knowledge about the association between diseases and symptoms and this knowledge.

Empirical knowledge can be acquired by a DSS in one of two general approaches. The first is a so-called top-down approach, wherein a domain expert "tells" the system how he thinks. The INTERNIST-1 and MYCIN programs were designed with this model. An alternative, "bottom-up," approach is

increasingly prevalent and made possible by new software tools and large databases (see Chap. 19). In this case, knowledge is automatically acquired by a DSS through analysis of a dataset. For example, a DSS may "learn" that heart rates greater than a certain number are associated with ST segment depression in a particular patient or patient population, or that hospitalization in a certain intensive care unit is associated with a high rate of central line infection (Fig. 11-12).

Top-down systems use rules, typically derived from experts. Bottom-up systems use tools like neural networks or machine learning in which "smart" software can find novel or unexpected information by analyzing large datasets for associations. Top-down systems typically require on-going maintenance and supervision, whereas bottom-up systems can be self-teaching.

Decision Support Logic

Decision support system engines use different combinations of reasoning, explanatory, and learning approaches. Mathematical models can be used to describe the interaction of dose and effect, such as the use of pharmacokinetic models relating to the administration of certain drugs. For example, a pharmacokinetic model might be used by a DSS to recommend the appropriate dose and dosing interval for a course of gentamicin in a patient of a known weight with a specific creatinine clearance.

Statistical methods are typically inductive, and based on the relationship of known antecedents (i.e., signs or symptoms) to an outcome (i.e., a diagnosis). The system is given the values of the antecedents for a specific patient (i.e., neck stiffness = TRUE, photophobia = TRUE) and produces an outcome (i.e., probability of meningitis) for that patient. This approach can be applied to diagnosis, prognosis, or therapeutic approach. Bayesian networks or "belief" networks fall into this category, and rely on Bayesian logic.

We have already discussed expert systems, which are intended to reproduce the thinking process taken by a "domain expert" in a specific area (such as infectious disease). The expert thinking processes are usually represented by a series of rules intended to express the way that the expert analyzes a

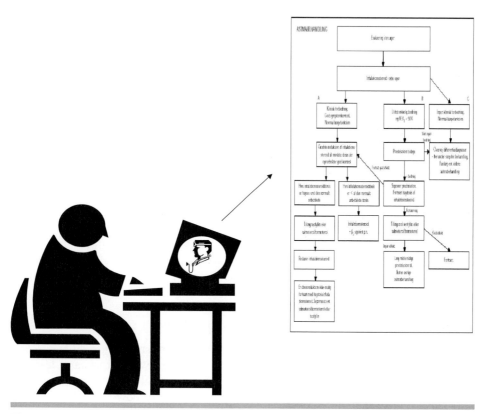

Figure 11-10
Strategy management decision support systems guide clinicians in the care of patients using consensus-based protocols or pathways.

problem, and can therefore "explain" their thinking, if asked. This explanatory capability is attractive because clinicians are understandably wary of solutions when they don't understand the derivation. A major downside for expert systems is the degree to which they need to be maintained as new knowledge emerges. Additionally, it has become clear that true experts arrive at conclusions using an associative or intuitive process that is not readily translated into effective rule sets.

Decision Support Modes

A DSS acts in one of three broad ways. Passive systems are given input with an implicit request for a response (Fig. 11-13). The MYCIN and INTERNIST-1 systems worked in this way. A passive

DSS can act as a consultant system or act to critique the performance of a clinician.

Semiactive systems sit in the background and prompt with reminders to act. A semiactive system might remind that an inoculation is due (i.e., DPT), list contraindications to a drug prescription or enumerate steps in a best-practice protocol. Semiactive systems can also be used to monitor physiologic variables such as heart rate and blood pressure, and alert clinicians about threshold-based or trend-based alarms (Fig. 11-14).

Finally, active DSSs can intervene automatically. An active DSS might order therapies (i.e., from a previously determined best-practice protocol) or investigations autonomously. Active systems could also be used to control the titration of a drug (such as an antihypertensive agent) based on a feedback

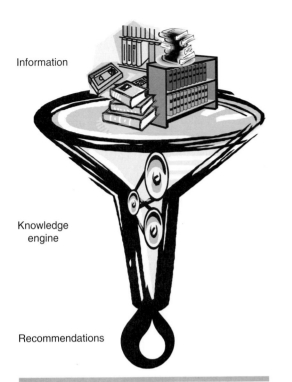

Information

Knowledge engine

Recommendations

Figure 11-11
Decision support system require an information base and an "engine" in order to make recommendations.

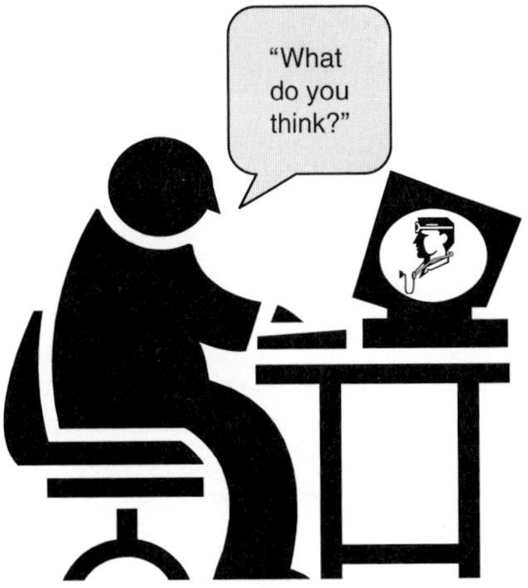

"What do you think?"

Figure 11-13
Passive DSSs wait to be asked before giving advice.

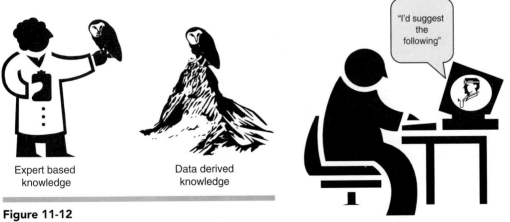

Expert based knowledge

Data derived knowledge

Figure 11-12
Expert (top-down) knowledge systems rely on preconstructed rules, whereas data derived (bottom-up) systems make use of the "mountains" of data that we now collect electronically.

"I'd suggest the following"

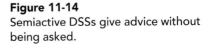

Figure 11-14
Semiactive DSSs give advice without being asked.

control loop or manage the weaning of mechanical ventilation. "Smart" DSSs have been integrated into newer pacemakers and implanted defibrillators to actively control the timing and dose of DC cardioversion (Fig. 11-15).

Implementation Issues

Key Points

- Clinicians *must* "buy-in" to a DSS in order to be comfortable using them, since they bear the ultimate responsibility for their actions.
- Issues include both the currency and accuracy of the knowledge base as well as the "truth" of the logical engine.
- Technical issues such as the way in which it performs with differing numbers of users, its response time.
- Clinician buy-in will depend to a large extent on the degree to which they were involved in the development of site-specific protocols.
- DSSs raise a variety of interesting medical-legal issues.

Some of the general implementation issues include quality, safety, and the use of standards across systems such as a uniform medical terminology. The quality and safety issue relates to the fact that, by adopting the recommendations of a DSS, the clinician is acting under the presumption that the recommendation is both accurate and safe. As with any system requiring maintenance, the potential for errors exists, and it is the clinician who bears the legal responsibility for orders written in his name. Clinicians will therefore need to be comfortable with the knowledge base and logic of a DSS in order to use it (Fig. 11-16).

The questions relating to the content of the knowledge base and rules of a DSS include: whether the knowledge bases have been accurately translated into the electronic format needed by the system, whether the knowledge has been peer-reviewed, whether the rules generated by the system have undergone peer-review, the currency of the information and how frequently it has been updated.

There are additional issues pertaining to the design aspects of a DSS such as the success with which it scales up with increased numbers of users. For example, a critical care physiologic monitoring DSS designed to alert when a patient's heart rate or blood pressure deviate may perform well with 10 patients, but degrade with larger numbers. While systems questions of this kind fall under the aegis of software quality control and

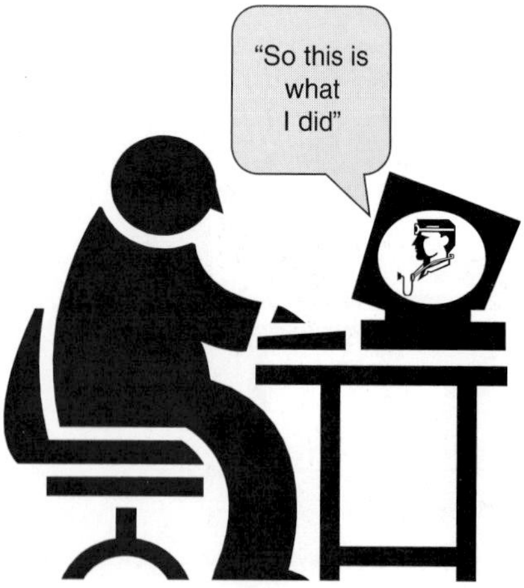

Figure 11-15
Active DSSs act without being asked.

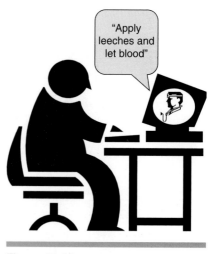

Figure 11-16
DSS logic and recommendations must be trustworthy to be accepted.

design, the consequences of poor programming may not become apparent until a system is tested under load in a clinical setting.

The terminology problem is common to any computerized medical system. There are a number of competing medical terminologies such as SNOMED, ICD9, and so on. While it is possible to map diagnoses from one terminology to another, there isn't a one-for-one equivalence and the adoption of a national-level, uniform technology is clearly desirable.

It is axiomatic that poorly designed software will be poorly accepted. However, it is also possible to imagine a system that is well maintained and has excellent software logic, but a poor user-interface. To be successful, DSSs must be deployed at the point of care, be easy to learn to use, and self-explanatory. Systems that increase the productivity of a clinician will be successful, whereas systems that are difficult to use and slow performance will fail. Integration of decision support tools into hand-held devices and familiar web-browsers facilitates acceptance.

Another critical aspect to the enthusiasm with which a system will be embraced in a medical community relates to the way in which it is deployed. Clinicians are far more likely to accept systems in which they feel a sense of ownership. For example, the inclusion of clinicians in the development process prior to deployment can identify local cultural issues that may impede acceptance. The designation of a local "champion" during deployment can reduce resistance to a system that might otherwise appear to be imposed from without.

DSSs can be used to provide continuing medical education, which is of growing importance as recertification increasingly becomes the norm. Alerts that permit the clinician to electively pursue the rationale or literature behind a recommended course of action will be welcomed. Systems that provide automatic feedback about proposed treatments will likely be accepted if they are not perceived to have a "big brother" flavor.

Specifically addressing the medico-legal aspects of DSSs, it is clear that the body of law informing many of the relevant issues has not yet been developed. The degree to which liability comes in play clearly relates to the degree of deviation from normal practice. Passive systems (as described above) are presumably less likely to increase or inherently create liability than active ones; for example, it is not clear to whom liability should be assigned in the event that an infusion delivered by a feedback-control loop system causes harm.

Some of the many legal questions that come to mind are: (1) to what degree is the clinician liable for harm due to a flaw in the DSS, (2) what if the clinician misuses the DSS, (3) what is the legal responsibility of the DSS vendor and to what extent does the contract between the vendor and the purchaser address it, and (4) what happens if a clinician is forced to work with a faulty DSS purchased by the health system in which he is employed (Fig. 11-17)? Another wrinkle relates to the clinician's liability should he choose to not follow the recommendations of a DSS. Is a clinician at greater risk for deferring to incorrect recommendations from a DSS or ignoring correct ones? It is obvious that there is the potential for tension between clinical judgment and decision support-based recommendations, much as any two clinicians may disagree about the correct course or sequence of actions. Furthermore, as DSSs achieve greater acceptance, clinicians' reliance on them will grow as will, presumably, their tendency to blindly accept recommendations.

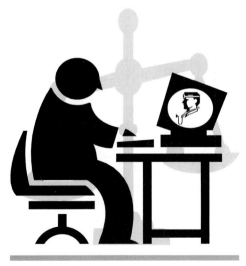

Figure 11-17
It is unclear where legal liability lies when a clinician follows advice from a DSS.

Summary

When asked, clinicians have identified a list of desired functions of DSSs, most of which are well within the capabilities of existing DSS software. They wish to have automatic order parsing using rules based on consensus guidelines from national medical societies, and the ability to electively request the relevant date of issue and derivation for a particular recommendation. This is promising in that it suggests a willingness on the part of clinicians to move toward consensus-based medicine, a goal that has been elusive in previous eras.

Clinicians also wish to have all relevant information derived from various patient care activities presented more or less concurrently, rather than having to open separate systems (i.e., windows). This includes information entered into and provided by the DSS.

Clinicians also want alerts generated by the DSS to cover a wide range of factors, including known allergies, patient-specific information (i.e., alerts tailored to the patient with breast cancer regarding new trials for which she might be eligible). In addition, the clinician wants to have access to the knowledge rules associated both with the condition and the interventions proposed by the DSS. This permits the clinician to evaluate the evidence underpinning the DSS rules.

Clinicians want prompts and reminders to engage in patient-specific preventative actions and reminders pertaining to actions that are underway (i.e., to follow up on a scheduled test or laboratory study). Acting in this way, DSSs facilitate patient care in an increasingly complex and fast-paced environment, which will enhance clinician buy-in.

Clinicians also want access to diagnostic support at the relevant point of their interaction with the EHR, CPOE, or DSS. This may come in the form of a simple list of the symptoms, signs, and expected laboratory findings associated with a specific diagnosis under consideration or by a more elaborate, smart diagnostic system along the lines of QMR, MYCIN, or DxPlain, as described above. Additionally, the DSS could act in either a passive or active role in suggesting diagnostic alternatives.

Clinicians want to be able to measure their own practice against that of peers (although they don't necessarily want that measurement done by employers or insurers). Potential comparison peer groups include other clinicians in a practice, institution, or specialty. This kind of peer group comparison can be useful in determining a clinician's efficiency, cost-effectiveness, and degree of compliance with standards of practice. Finally, clinicians may wish to perform concurrent or retrospective audits of individual aspects of their practice.

As the tools desired by clinicians become more generally available, nonintrusive, and easy to use by clinicians, they will insinuate themselves into practice routines. Decision support applications will grow in scope as new hardware and software tools become available, and as the acceptability of DSSs in medical practice are demonstrated. A useful comparison can be made to the aviation industry, in which current generation commercial cockpits have become highly automated and airplanes are flown "by wire." Military aviation and aviation research is even further ahead as are many of the tools used in battlefield analysis, command, and control. As with these other applications, medicine is a technology rich environment, but it has been much slower to automate and delegate tasks to computers and software. The rapidly growing price and efficiency pressures on the medical industry will, by necessity, increase the rate of change and the speed of adoption of decision support tools.

Suggested Readings

Ball MJ, Berner E. *Clinical Decision Support Systems: Theory and Practice*. Springer, 1998.

Teich JM, Wrinn MM. *Clinical Decision Support Systems Come of Age*. MD Computing Jan/Feb 2000, pp. 43–46. rhttp://www.ahrq.gov/clinic/ptsafety/chap53.htm.

Kaushal R, Bates DW. Computerized Physician Order Entry (CPOE) with Clinical Decision Support Systems (CDSSs). In: Tierney WM (ed.), *Evidence Report/Technology Assessment No. 43, Making Health Care Safer: A Critical Analysis of Patient Safety Practices*. AHRQ Publication No. 01-E058, 2001, pp. 59–69.

Email

Introduction

Key Points

- Email has many appealing features as a form of communication in the medical setting.
- Email can be used to communicate between providers and patients or from provider to provider.

The American Medical Informatics Association, which has taken a lead role in defining the issues associated with email in the medical setting, defines patient-provider email as "computer-based communication between clinicians and patients within a contractual relationship in which the health care provider has taken on an explicit measure of responsibility for the client's care." There are wide ranges of issues inherent in email communications between a clinician and a patient. Consider the email shown in Fig. 12-1. Provider-provider patient-related email is not encompassed in this definition, but raises some of the same issues.

A third kind of communication is email from a provider to a "client" with whom there is no contractual relationship. There are, for example, web sites, newsgroups, and discussion groups wherein a clinician undertakes to provide medical advice in the absence of a traditionally defined medical role. One example of a relatively successful site of this type is MyDoc.com, which provides web-based medical advice (in some states). This chapter will deal primarily with patient-provider and provider-provider email.

Medical Email

Key Points

- Email's advantages include its ability to uncouple the communications of the two parties so that they don't need to be at two ends of a phone line but can communicate more quickly than letters permit.
- Email can be used for f/u, reinforcement, amplification, or education.
- Email's disadvantages include its similarity to a conversation but lack of the usual cues which permits ambiguous or disinhibited communications.
- Email is also relatively insecure and therefore problematic for medical communications.
- Email has advantages and disadvantages that are unique and differ from those of other medical communication formats.

Advantages of Email Communication

Email is well suited to the kinds of communication that are likely to occur between a provider and a patient or a peer. For example, it is asynchronous and therefore doesn't require the simultaneous presence of both parties. This is ideal for busy physicians and other healthcare providers, who are not typically deskbound and are often difficult to reach (Fig. 12-2).

Email is less formal than a letter (and less expensive) but more permanent and typically more structured than a phone conversation. It is equally well suited to the exchange of a quick question and answer, and more complicated interaction.

```
✉ unhappy in Seattle - Message (Rich Text)              _ □ ✗
 File  Edit  View  Insert  Format  Tools  Actions  Help
 ▣ Send  🖫 🖨  ✂ 📋  📎  🔖✓  📇 Options...  »  Arial        ▾  A  B  I  U  ⇇ »
```

To...	Dr. John Doe
Cc...	
Bcc...	
Subject:	unhappy in Seattle

```
I feel as if I can trust you, and I don't know where else
to turn. I have moved to Seattle in the last couple of
weeks and left my husband. I thought this would be a
solution, but it only seems to have made things worse. My
family has turned against me since they learned about the
AIDS test, and I feel as if I have nowhere to turn. I
think constantly about taking a lot of those pills you
prescribed for me and just going to sleep. What should I
do?
```

Figure 12-1
Example of an email that raises many issues about privacy, malpractice, response time, and licensure.

Email is also an excellent format for follow-up communication after an office visit, and can be used for reinforcement, amplification, or provision of additional information not available at the time of the visit (i.e., lab or pathology results). Preformatted material (educational material about diseases, instructions regarding medications or wound care, and so on) can be attached to an email or formatted as an email. Automatic hyperlinks to other resources on the Internet (web sites, newsgroups, and so on) are readily included in most email clients. Email messages can be stored electronically or in a paper format to retain a "paper trail" documenting what has been communicated by whom and when.

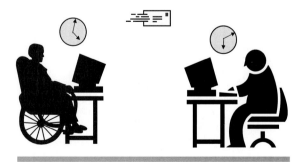

Figure 12-2
Email permits efficient communication between two parties who are unlinked in time, unlike the phone.

Disadvantages of Email Communication

The disadvantages of the use of email as a communication tool are inextricably intertwined with its advantages. Its informality relative to a letter and the lack of the cues inherent to verbal communication (in person or on a phone) make email

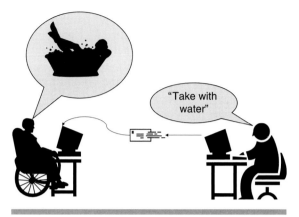

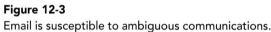

Figure 12-3
Email is susceptible to ambiguous communications.

susceptible to miscommunication (Fig. 12-3). For example, one might not choose to say "take that with a grain of salt" to some patients for fear that they might. Sarcasm and wit are frequently misinterpreted in email.

Anger or frustration can be expected occasionally in email from patients to providers and should be treated in the same dispassionate fashion that providers would use in dealing with patients expressing those same emotions directly. All correspondence pertaining to patient care issues is both discoverable in the legal sense and able to be discovered after deletion from a local computer.

Electronic messages can be recovered because of the unique properties of email. Like a letter or postcard, email passes from an originating local machine through virtual post offices to a destination machine. Unlike "snail mail," however, email messages leave copies of themselves at the post offices. This occurs because data are backed-up on the intermediary systems so that they can be reconstituted in the event of a catastrophic failure (Fig. 12-4).

Email Authentication and Encryption

The best way to preserve the advantages of email communication and protect against its shortcomings is email encryption. The Healthcare Insurance Portability and Accountability Act (HIPAA) requires that online communications regarding patient care (between a provider and patient, or among providers) be conducted securely with provisions for

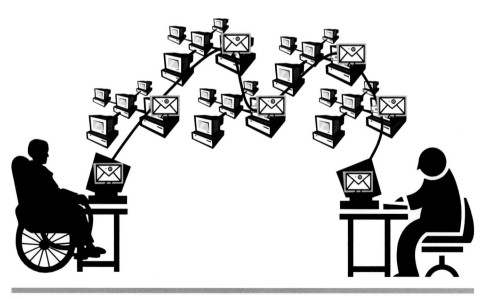

Figure 12-4
Email leaves copies of itself on many computers.

Table 12-1   Security definitions

HIPAA electronic data interchange requirements	
Encryption	Encryption of email and other patient data to protect information from unauthorized access
Authentication	Ensuring that the parties at both ends of EDI are who they say they are
Audit trails	Maintenance of a record of who accessed what information when
Authorization	Ensuring that the parties involved in EDI are allowed to do what they do with patient health information

encryption and authentication of the parties at both ends of the exchange (Table 12-1).

Powerful encryption software is available from a number of providers, although encryption is not yet built into most email client programs. The progenitor algorithm is known as pretty good privacy (PGP). Another widely used encryption system is the secure/multipurpose Internet mail extensions (S/MIME). Both systems use strong encryption.

Strong encryption techniques can be used to guarantee important components of a transaction between a provider and a patient, including the authenticity of the sender, the privacy of the communication, and the time of the communication. These techniques rely on a combination of a publicly available key, a private key known only to you or your computer and an authenticating approach intended to ensure that each party in a transaction is who they say they are (Fig. 12-5).

Using cryptographic techniques, electronic communications can be encrypted, "indelibly" time stamped, digitally signed, made tamper proof and nonrepudiable. Time stamping ensures the accurate timing and sequencing of orders, data entries, or communications (Fig. 12-6).

The utility of a digital signature is obvious. It can be used to guarantee the signature on a medical order or prescription (Fig. 12-7).

Tamper-proofing or content validation ensures the integrity of communications between providers or patients and providers (Fig. 12-8). One can imagine situations in which a hostile individual might wish alter the content or intent of a message between

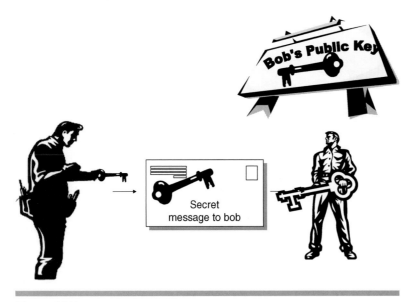

Figure 12-5
Public key/private key encryption: Joe sends Bob a message encrypted with Bob's public key and Bob decrypts with his private key.

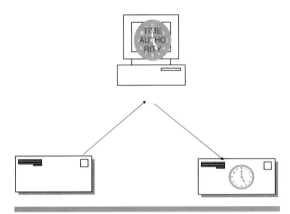

Figure 12-6
A time stamping authority certifies the contents of
a document at the time it receives it.

a provider and a patient. Tamper-proofing prevents
this.

Finally, by eliminating the possibility that a party
could deny (repudiate) having sent an email (i.e., prescription), the integrity of email as a legal document
is ensured, which is essential to its acceptance as integral part of medical practice (Fig. 12-9).

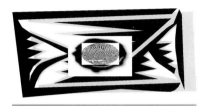

Figure 12-8
Tamper-proofing is assured using a
digital seal.

Many of the major medical societies and malpractice insurers recommend that all online communications between providers and their patients should be
encrypted both to preserve privacy and confidentiality as well as to reduce liability (Chap. 15). Key web
sites are listed below:

American Academy of Family Practice
    Recommendations (http://www.aafp.org/x452.xml)

American Medical Association Recommendations
    (http://www.ama-assn.org/ama/pub/category/2386.html)

American Medical Informatics Association Recommendations
    (http://www.amia.org/pubs/other/email_guidelines.html)

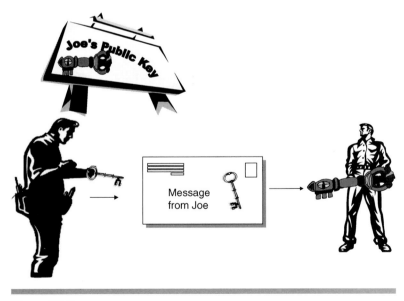

Figure 12-7
Document encrypted/signed with Joe's private key: if his public key
decrypts it, it came from Joe.

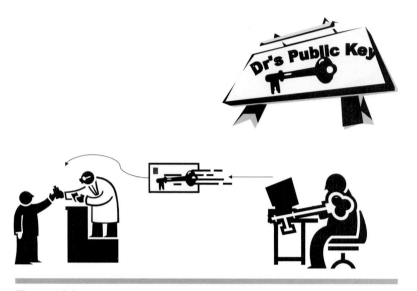

Figure 12-9
A prescription can be digitally signed and encrypted by an MD, sent over the Internet and cannot be repudiated.

Email among providers is often confined to a site, i.e., an academic medical center, and therefore conducted behind the protective screen of a firewall. These emails do not travel across the Internet and are not necessarily subject to the usual requirements for encryption and authentication (Fig. 12-10).

Email Communication Guidelines

Historically, communications between patient and provider have been limited to face to face encounters,

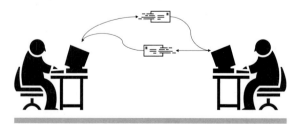

Figure 12-10
Provider-provider email can be used for patient care communications if confined within a HIPAA compliant intranet.

telephone exchanges, or letters. These traditional approaches will be preferable to many patients who are unfamiliar with or leery of email. Conversely, others will prefer email communications wherever possible. A recent study by Medem (a healthcare consortium made up of leading medical societies) showed that the volume of physician-patient email tripled over the year ending in May 2001. Patients want to be able to use email for various services, and more than half of the patients surveyed in one study indicated that they would be willing to switch to a physician who provides these services by email (Fig. 12-11).

These data suggest that providers will inevitably use email communications in their practices in various ways. So-called "early-adopters" of new technology have already integrated email into their practices. However, the majority of practitioners haven't yet done so, and the way in which they do will be to some degree dependent on the nature of their practice (solo vs. group), and the ease with which email is integrated into their patient management.

Practitioners who function in a large, integrated system such as an academic medical center will most

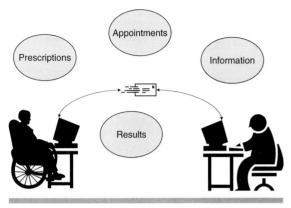
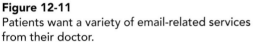

Figure 12-11
Patients want a variety of email-related services from their doctor.

likely be provided with email services that meet all regulatory requirements and adhere to standards defined by the system's computer administrators. Solo and small group practitioners will be more likely to purchase email and web services from intermediary providers who act, in effect, as medically oriented Internet service providers (ISPs). Medem is an example of a business that provides secure messaging for communications between patients and providers or from one provider to another. These communications are encrypted and meet regulatory requirements for security and privacy.

Several medical associations have developed recommendations about email communication between providers and patients. Thease communications can be thought of as a contract meeting the following set of expectations:

- All email should be encrypted
- Correspondents should be authenticated (guarantee you are who you say you are)
- Patient confidentiality should be protected
- Unauthorized access to email (electronic or paper) should be prevented
- Patient should provide informed consent regarding the scope and nature of electronic communications
- Electronic communications should (ideally) occur in the context of a preexisting doctor-patient relationship

- Online communications are to be considered a part of the patient's medical record and should be included with same

Many organizations recommend that the patient and physician sign an agreement formalizing their expectations of email communication. The recommended elements of that contract are detailed in Table 12-2.

There are specific ways in which email can be used in medical communication from (Fig. 12-12):

- A provider to a patient:
  - Prescription refills
  - Lab results reporting
  - Appointment reminders
  - Insurance questions
  - Follow-up inquiries

- A provider to groups of patients:
  - Information pertaining to general health information (i.e., new dietary recommendations for all patients)
  - Information to specific patient groups (i.e., new mammogram guidelines)
  - Staffing or coverage changes (e.g., the hiring of a new provider or change in provider availability)

- A patient to a provider:
  - Inform primary about visits to other physicians or new issues
  - Ask questions
  - Upload measurements from home medical devices such as blood pressure or glucose measurements

Patient lists should be suppressed when email is sent from a provider to a group of patients (which can be done by addressing the email to oneself and using the "blind cc:" line for the intended addressees). Bulk communications are facilitated by the creation and maintenance of patient lists (such as "all patients," "hypertensive patients," "female patients born 50 years go," and so on) (Fig. 12-13).

All incoming email from patients should be responded to, automatically if possible as in (Fig. 12-14).

Table 12-2   Communication guidelines

Issue	Recommendation
Email turnaround	Establish expected response time. Do not use email for urgent issues
Privacy	Clarify who will have access to patient email and that it is included in the record
Email management	Patient should know who handles email when addressee is there and when away
Paper trail	Paper copies of all emails should beplaced in medical record
Transaction	Clarify what kinds of problems (prescriptions, routine questions) and content (nonsensitive material) can behandled by email
Format	Clarify how patient should title (subject line) and identify (name, clinic ID) email
Identification	Patient's name and medical recordnumber should be included in email toclinician
	The clinician's name, contact info, andalternative contact approaches shouldbe a part of outgoing email
Email confirmation	Patient and provider should confirm receipt of all emails using autoreply
	Send new email to indicate completion of request
Archive and retrieval	Clinicians should develop email archival and retrieval mechanisms
Distribution lists	Clinician should develop various distribution lists of patients as appropriate, but should not send group mailings where recipient lists are visible (use blind copy feature)
Emotion	Avoid anger, sarcasm, criticism, and libelous references to third parties in email
Escalation	The patient should be advised when and how to escalate issues initially dealt with in email
Consent	Develop informed consent document covering communication expectations, encryption, indemnification, and so on
Encryption	Provider and patient expectations and capabilities pertaining to encryption of email should be detailed when appropriate
Content	Patients should be reminded to keep messages concise
	Patients should be told when they violate guidelines
	Clinician may terminate email communications with patients who repeatedly violate guidelines

The response indicates that the message was received and provides instructions for alternative contact if necessary. Email should be archived (stored) and copies of correspondence should be placed in the chart. When action is necessary, such as the refilling of a prescription, an email should be sent to the patient confirming completion of the action.

Site Management

In addition to the policies pertaining to provider-patient communication, an additional set of policies must be defined pertaining to administrative management of email at the provider's end. Issues include the designation of who (clerical vs. provider)

will triage email, how often will email be checked, who will print and file email messages, how and how frequently will archiving be performed, and when and how encryption will be used in patient-provider email.

Another set of considerations pertains to the "architecture" of the providers' email accounts. One approach to the organization of incoming email is to divide it by topic (i.e., billingquestion @doctors.clinic). An alternative approach is to require the patient to specify the topic of the email in the subject line of the email and direct it to the provider. Providers will need to determine whether or not any, some, or all patient will have access to their provider-specific email accounts.

Consideration should be given to the location and visibility of terminal screens and printers used

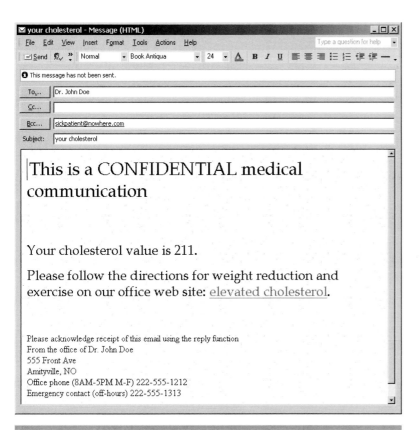

Figure 12-12
Example of results sent to a patient by email.

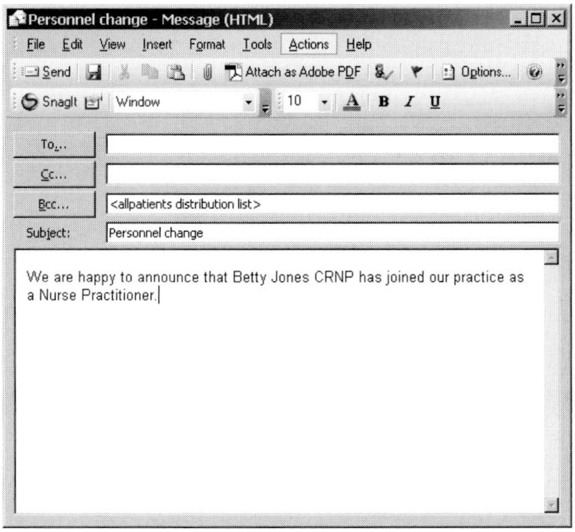

Figure 12-13
Example of a bulk email sent to all patients.

for email management—patient-provider email content should not be visible to patients or clinic personnel not directly involved in email management. Terminals used for email management should be equipped with password-protected screensavers that are automatically invoked after a brief period of inactivity. Ideally, an audit trail should be established indicating who accessed what email when. Antiviral packages that automatically screen incoming and outgoing email and are automatically updated with new antiviral definitions should be installed on appropriate personal computers.

Those decisions which are codified as policies by the provider should be specified as such and included in the provider's paper and/or electronic policy manual. Clinic employees should be familiar

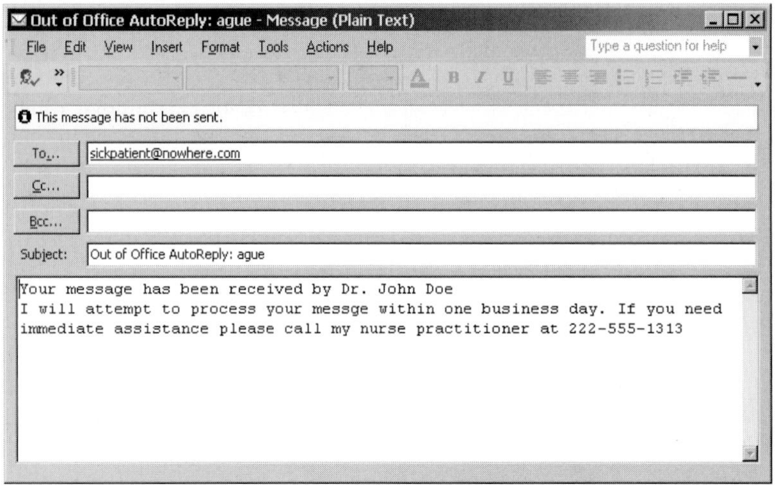

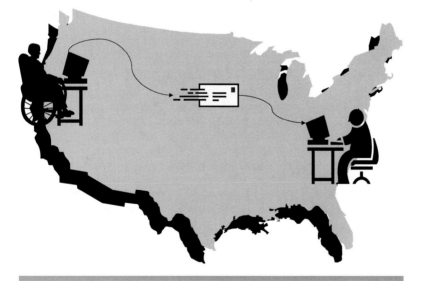

Figure 12-14
Example of an automatic reply on receipt of an email.

Figure 12-15
Email coming from out of state may pose specific legal issues.

with the policies and held accountable to them (Table 12-3).

Medico-Legal Considerations

There is insufficient case law to elucidate many of the legal issues pertaining to email-related responsibilities. Areas of obvious interest and concern are those pertaining to data security and provider liability. It is important to emphasize some of the differences between traditional patient-provider communication and email when talking about liability. Email messages often travel over the Internet using ad hoc routes.

Some practices using email have implemented protective approaches such as "click-through" messages reading "By clicking this button, you acknowledge that you are patient X." Alternatively, or complementarily, some providers have required patients to present themselves with a legal form of ID to authenticate their email address. These practices represent efforts to ensure the identity of the individual with whom they are communicating.

One troublesome aspect of online communications is that they can cross state lines transparently. One might, for example, send an email to a patient without having any clue as to their location, which might be in an adjacent state in which the provider is not licensed. Because these communications are currently subject to the requirements of state licensure, they may increase risk to a provider (Fig. 12-15). A conservative approach would be to:

- Ascertain the physical location of a patient prior to communicating about diagnosis or treatment.

- If the patient is not in a state in which the provider is licensed, communications should be limited to administrative (i.e., scheduling) issues.

It is quite possible that a hostile intermediary, who is not bound to confidentiality agreements, could gain access to those communications. Because of these concerns and the fact that the laws and landscape of medical email are changing rapidly, most practitioners will choose to manage their email communications with the assistance of a third party (such as a hospital information system or a medical ISP).

Billing for electronic communications

Third party payers are increasingly willing to consider reimbursement for electronic communications. They will undoubtedly require compliance with documentary and behavioral standards

Table 12-3 Exemplar email policies

Issue	Recommendation
Agreement with patient	Develop email specific informed consent and place in medical record
Consent components	Terms of communication described in Table 12-2
	Escalation instructions
	Describe security mechanisms in place
	Hold healthcare institution harmless for information lost due to technical failures
	Waive encryption requirements at patient's insistence
Security policies	Never forward patient's information without their consent
	Use password-protected screensaver
	Never use patient info in marketing effort
	Ensure clinician's professional email not accessible by clinician's family members
	Do not use wireless communications for patient info unless encryption in place
	Double check all to:/cc:/bcc: fields prior to transmission of email
	Perform weekly or more frequent email back-ups onto long-term storage using standards for paper medical records
	Commit policies to written and electronic format

including informed consent, fee disclosure, appropriate billing (i.e., for evaluation and management rather than scheduling or prescribing).

Conclusion

Email is not yet a standard component of medical communications, but it is certain to become so. While the regulatory, legal, and reimbursement aspects are changing rapidly, a consensus has developed about a number of the key aspects of email in a medical setting. As a result, even a technically unsophisticated provider can comfortably engage in some forms of medically oriented communication with peers or patients under the aegis of an "umbrella" organization providing mechanisms for encryption and authentication or a secure, enclosed messaging environment.

Suggested Readings

Guidelines for the Clinical Use of Electronic Mail with Patients. http://www.amia.org/pubs/other/email_guidelines.html.
Guidelines for Physician-Patient Electronic Communications. http://www.ama-assn.org/ama/pub/category/2386.html.

13 Internet and Medicine

Introduction

Key Points

- Health information is increasingly available on the Internet and "pushed" through portals.
- Internet medical information may be presented with hidden biases or be inaccurate.
- Until standards are developed, the principle of caveat emptor (buyer beware) is best followed.

Whereas patients may once have thought of medical knowledge as the sole province of its priests and priestesses—doctors and nurses, the advent of the Internet and ready access to medical information has radically changed things. Every news magazine has run a story on patients or parents who have exhaustively searched the Internet for obscure medical information. All of the major news portals now have a section dedicated to health stories and, as a result, more health information is available to patients than ever before.

Every office-based practitioner has dealt with new patients who arrive with a fistful of information pertaining to their medical problem. Patients are increasingly well informed or at least attempt to be so, and they have the vast resources of the Internet at their disposal (Fig. 13-1). There is much to be said for having more well-informed patients, but it has become clear that much of the medical information on the Internet is placed there for some form of secondary gain.

Clinicians have also come to rely on the Internet for medical information, and while they may be more savvy or skeptical consumers, they are subject to the same biases and inaccuracies as patients in some of the information they find. There are growing efforts by the government and professional organizations to create certifications or "seals of approval" indicating that the content on a health information site is accurate and current (Fig. 13-2).

Internet Usage by Patients

Key Points

- One of the key uses of the Internet is to search for medical information.
- While there are medical search engines, medical content is largely presented "as is."

There are an estimated 20,000 or more websites on the Internet dedicated to every kind of health information. Some studies have shown that between 50 and 80% of adults with Internet access use it for medical purposes; in fact, a recent Harris survey estimated that 97 million adults have used the Internet to look for health-related materials. More than 70% of the people who look for medical information on the Web use it to assist in their medical decision-making. Patients search for drug and disease information as well as providers. The Internet has already had a significant effect on the practice of medicine and those impacts are likely to grow as the percentage of the population with Internet access and computer facility increases.

Patients who scan the Internet for medical information are confronted with an enormous quantity of material: the Internet is the largest searchable repository of medical information in the world. The problem is that the information may be uninterpretable (Fig. 13-3), as in the case of many medical studies published in peer-reviewed journals, or wrong. There are medical search engines, but most

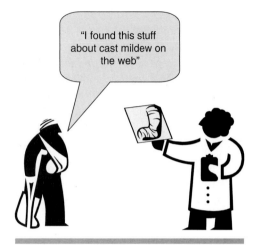

Figure 13-1
Patients do their own web-based research prior to office visits.

consumers use standard search engines, and may be naïve to the nuances of the search algorithms and resulting rankings. It is possible, for example, for a site to "game" the search engine in order to achieve a high ranking or to pay for same.

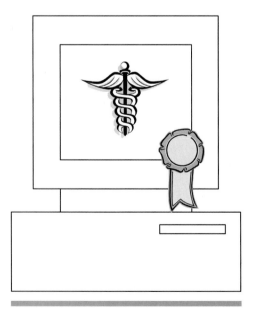

Figure 13-2
There is a growing need for a health-care-related web site "seal of approval."

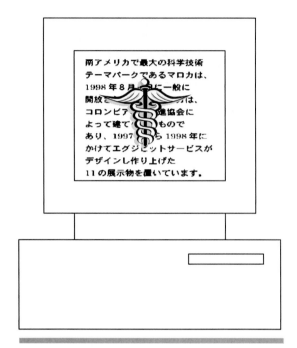

Figure 13-3
Web site health material may be confusing or uninterpretable to the average patient either because of medical jargonism or the reading grade level of the material is pitched too high.

Quality of Internet Medical Information

Key Points

- Internet medical information can come from reputable, nonaligned providers, from drug companies, from practitioners looking to sell their "product" or from fringe groups.

- Systematic evaluations of medical content on the web have found inaccurate, inconsistent information presented at a reading level too high for the average consumer.

- It is critical to evaluate the credentials of content providers to determine their qualifications and the degree to which the information on the site might be biased.

- Medical hucksterism is rampant and the FTC and FDA have begun to prosecute egregious cases.

While the amount of medical information on the Internet increases exponentially, the quality of that information is variable. In many senses, current day Internet medical information harkens back to the era of medicine prior to the Flexner report, when hucksters and medical pedigree mills abounded. Spam pitches for various drugs and online pharmacies, websites with every imaginable medical theme, and glossy "brochure" web sites from plastic surgery vendors are the modern day equivalents of snake oil sales. To be fair, there are a variety of credible medical sites as well (Fig. 13-4).

Professional societies and disease-specific organizations usually have information for patients pertaining to that field. Several academic institutions have developed excellent general information sites for patients covering a variety of medical topics. Drug companies have drug-specific information, although these sites are typically developed with an ulterior motive, i.e., enhanced sales of that drug.

A few commercial organizations have aggregated a variety of medical resources including information for patients.

A number of studies have been done to evaluate health information on the Internet with the general theme of quality including accuracy, completeness, readability, design, and referencing. Most have concluded that quality is a problem. Problem areas include the presentation of inaccurate or inconsistent information, information pitched at the wrong reading level (i.e., out of reach of the general web readership), failure to declare a potential bias (i.e., web site sponsored by a drug company), and so some have proposed the creation of rating systems or quality designations (such as a "seal of approval").

Literature

In response to concerns about the quality of health information on the Internet, the California

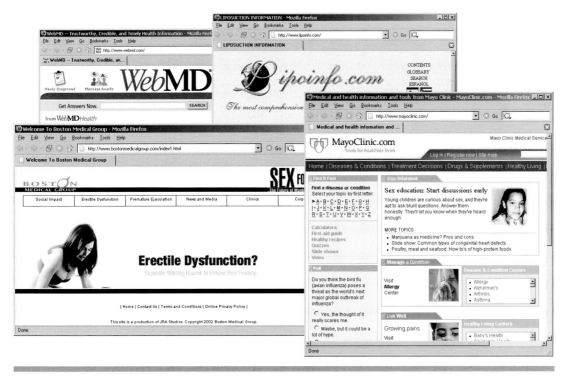

Figure 13-4
There are a variety of medically oriented sites with differing missions and agendas on the Internet.

Healthcare Foundation commissioned the Rand Corporation to do a large study describing and evaluating English and Spanish health information on the Internet which was published in the Journal of the American Medical Association in 2001. The study addressed three major questions. The first was what type of condition-specific information is identified by search engines and how efficiently they find same. The second pertained to the accuracy, comprehensiveness, and currency of the information. The third related to the level of literacy required by the consumer to understand the information presented on the web site.

The study focused on four common medical conditions: breast cancer, childhood asthma, depression, and obesity. It evaluated information from English and Spanish language web sites. The rationale for the choice of conditions was the fact that they affect diverse populations and are associated with disability and early death (Table 13-1).

The searches were performed on 10 English and 4 Spanish search engines, used standardized searches and simple search terms. The second phase of the study evaluated a number of English and Spanish language sites in terms of the degree to which they answered key questions about each of the diseases of interest. The questions were meant to reflect the kind of information that consumers are likely to seek (i.e., patient concerns) and the kind of information that information providers should offer (i.e., key concepts). Finally these sites were evaluated for readability and the grade level of the information presented in the two languages.

The study resulted in a number of interesting and cautionary findings. Few of the searches found relevant health information: there was a 20% chance of

finding good information on English sites and a 10–15% chance on Spanish sites. The search engines presented disparate results when presented with the same search terms. This is not a surprise to most users of the Web, but suggests an underlying bias that skews the responses of the search engines in one direction or another. The information on medical web sites is quite commercialized—much of the information is promotional and not necessarily clearly identified as such. A generic example might be a web site appearing to be primarily about the signs and symptoms of seasonal asthma that recommends treatment with a specific drug, where the web site is paid for and maintained by the drug company that sells the drug.

A second key finding of this study relates to the relative inconsistency of the information available on medical web sites. Important information was missing from many sites, information was out of date, information from one web site was internally inconsistent, coverage varied by topic and, not surprisingly, the comprehensiveness of topic coverage varied across web sites. For example, the information regarding breast cancer was quite good on cancer-related sites.

Finally, the study concluded that, while the average literacy level of most of the population is at the 9th grade reading level, most of the web sites were written at the college level. The obvious implication is that most health-related web sites present medical information one reading level above that of the portion of the population that most needs the information.

This study suggested that consumers beware of information on the web, both as it relates to accuracy and motivation. The authors suggested that consumer advocacy groups adopt or endorse a few high quality sites on particular topics and press for continual maintenance and improvement of the information presented on those sites. They suggested that health care professionals be cognizant of the benefits and pitfalls of web-based information and advocate for improved web content through professional and specialty societies. Web content providers were encouraged to subject their content to periodic expert review for the accuracy, currency, comprehensiveness, and readability of

Table 13-1 Disease information accuracy

	English (%)	Spanish (%)
Breast cancer	91	96
Asthma	84	53
Depression	75	63
Obesity	86	68

the content they provide. Finally policy makers and regulators were encouraged to attend to web health information, fund good sites, and fund efforts to evaluate the use of the web for health information mining.

Another recent *JAMA* study reported in 2002 attempted to define best-practice approaches to evaluating web-based health information. The authors evaluated about 80 manuscripts evaluating about 6000 web sites. They determined that most studies of web content defined the quality of the content by its accuracy, completeness, readability, design, disclosures, and provided references. As with the previously cited Rand study, the quality of web health content was found to be problematic. More importantly, these authors determined that a consistent and rigorous approach to the evaluation of web content is lacking. Fortunately, a common set of criteria for consumers to judge health care content on the web are beginning to emerge.

Quality Criteria for Web Sites

The old Roman adage *caveat emptor* clearly holds true for the online health content. There are a series of general recommendations that a clinician can make to patients. The first is that the choice of online health information providers should be handled to some extent like the choice of a doctor. It is reasonable and appropriate to get more than one opinion and compare them. Look for the information at an organization in which you have confidence—perhaps a well-known tertiary care center with a web site. Fortunately, it is less costly to "shop" for medical information on the web than it is to seek several separate medical opinions.

It is also very important to determine the credentials of the information source. Look for information relating to sponsorship of a web site. Pharmaceutical companies may pay for web sites promoting drugs through seemingly nonaligned "trusts." The absence of clear-cut contact information should raise an alarm. Web site content should be reviewed with an implicit question about the motivation of the authors or underwriters of a site (Fig. 13-5).

As with medical information provided by a clinician, medical web information is probably less credible if it is overly authoritative, definitive, or disparaging about alternatives. Look for the sources of content provided on the web site: is the content reviewed by an editorial board of experts, is it well referenced, is it up-to-date.

It is critical for patients to avoid filling out web forms with medical information unless the privacy of that information can be assured. Similarly, it is inappropriate to interact with a web-based "physician" proposing to diagnose and or treat based on a web interaction (Fig. 13-6).

The American Medical Association established a set of principles relating to the content of web sites they endorse. Their principles cover site content, advertising, privacy, and e-commerce. The AMA attempts to provide visitors to these sites with sites having clear-cut navigation, ownership disclosure, and information about what browsers are supported. The principles specify guidelines for editorial review relating to the process of review, the language complexity of the content, the date of posting, and sources of editorial content.

There are specifications describing intersite links and navigation, the use of intrasite navigation tools, and directions on downloading files (i.e., pdf documents or pictures) from the site. Advertising is permitted but should not be construed as endorsement by the AMA. Digital advertisements should be separated distinctly from editorial content. Sponsorship is also permitted provided it is acknowledged. Web site privacy and confidentiality policies prohibit the collection and dissemination of information about individual visitors to the site without their express, informed consent. In terms of e-commerce, the AMA principles require visitors to be informed about the use of encryption and security software during transactions.

Hucksterism

Health-related products and services have become a multi—billion-dollar business where products touting cures for chronic or terminal illnesses, discretionary surgical services and rejuvenation remedies are advertised on web sites, in chat rooms, and in

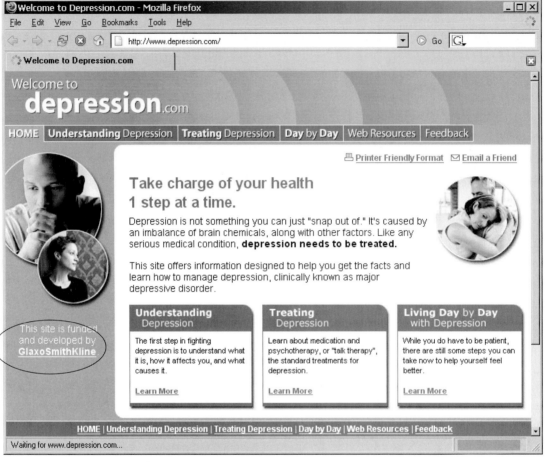

Figure 13-5
Web sites can have "hidden" agenda as in this site funded by a drug company.

unsolicited email. Some of the common chronic diseases targeted by hucksters include cancer, HIV, Alzheimer's, arthritis, multiple sclerosis, and diabetes (Fig. 13-7).

Online marketers can gain almost immediate, cheap access to a huge, international audience by marketing on the web. It is relatively inexpensive to create a web site or to fire off Spam. It is also relatively simple to embed terms in a web site that will draw desperate patients to the site. For example, by placing terms like "cancer therapy," "cancer treatment," or "cancer survivor" in a web site's text,

search engines will direct consumers seeking those terms to that site. Traditional marketing techniques for mass mailing can be used to design Spam that might engage the attention of consumers with specific health care problems or interests (Fig. 13-8).

The federal government, acting through the Food and Drug Administration and the Federal Trade Commission developed Operation Cure All in an effort to combat healthcare fraud, both on and off line. They have used a combination of prosecutions, public awareness, and education campaigns. Specific recommendations for

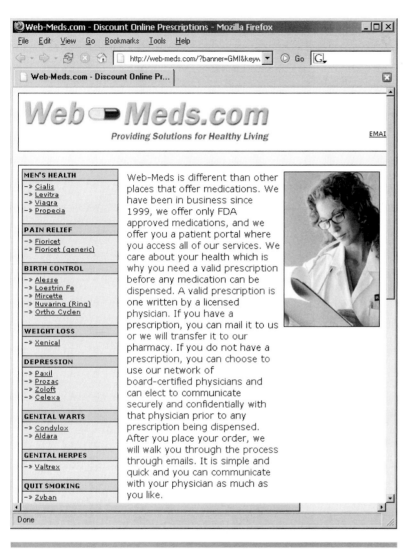

Figure 13-6
Site offering a network of physicians to "help" with prescriptions for narcotics, antidepressants, and drugs for erectile dysfunction.

consumers and patients include suggestions to beware of claims that a product is a "breakthrough," "cure-all," has a "secret ingredient," or is an "ancient remedy." Miracle stories of patients who took the advertised product are usually detail-laden and impossible to substantiate. They suggest that patients beware of claims that a specific product is available from a single source and that they will provide a money-back guarantee. Finally, the FTC warns against web sites failing to list a company's name, address, or other contact information. There are additional warnings about dietary supplements that are marketed as "natural" medicines, such as St. John's Wort, shark cartilage, ephedra, L-tryptophan, and so on.

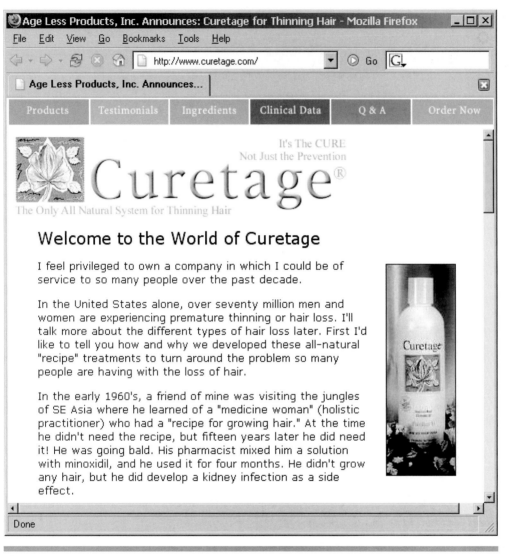

Figure 13-7
The Internet is rife with sites appealing to the naïve or desperate patient.

 Conclusion

The Internet will undoubtedly continue to grow as a medical reference resource and become a major vehicle for the delivery of healthcare through telemedicine applications. In the near-term, the appropriate uses of email communications between patients and physicians will become apparent, as will the reimbursement and legal ramifications. With the maturation of digital signatures and authentication, prescriptions will be handled by web-based communications. As multimedia tools such as microphones and cameras become more common, the appropriate uses of medical

VIAGRA - Message (HTML)

File   Edit   View   Insert   Format   Tools   Actions   Help

Send | 🔲 | ✂ 📋 📋 | 📎 | 🗐 Attach as Adobe PDF | &ᵥ | ! | ↓ | ❦ | | 🔲 Options... | @

🌀 SnagIt 🗐 | Window ...

To... | Anyone.at.all@world.com

Cc... |

Bcc... |

Subject: | VIAGRA

Hello!

Viagra is the #1 med to struggle with mens' erectile dysfunction.
Like one jokes sais, it is stronq enouqh for a man ,but made for a woman ;-)

Ordering Viagra online is a very convinient ,fast and secure way!
Millions of people do it daily to save their privacy and money

HYPERLINK "http://iabchkjlm.onlinewebmeds.info/?defgjlmxssryizgvabchk"Order
here...

Figure 13-8
Drug-related Spam is a growing nuisance.

multimedia presentations and communications will develop. Futurists have speculated about the emergence of a population of medical "guides" who could assist patients wishing to research a particular topic, treatment, or disease, relying on the guide to find reputable, balanced information.

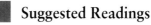 **Suggested Readings**

http://www.fda.gov/buyonline/.
http://www.fda.gov/cder/consumerinfo/
  Buy_meds_online_text.htm.
http://www.nlm.nih.gov/medlineplus/
  healthywebsurfing.html.

CHAPTER 14 — Telemedicine

Introduction

Key Points

▨ Telemedicine (or telehealth) is slowly gaining definition as a term describing a variety of approaches to healthcare using communications links.

▨ By removing the requirement for physical presence (of the patient, provider, or educator), telemedicine permits fundamental changes in health care delivery, administration, and education.

▨ Telemedicine has significant ramifications relating to licensure and malpractice that have yet to be fully defined.

Telemedicine and telehealth are two terms that are slowly creeping into public awareness. The former is a subset of the latter. Telehealth is the delivery of healthcare over a distance using tools such as the telephone, email, video, and computers. Patients who look to the Internet for information about healthcare are engaged in telehealth. Physicians who consult over the Internet are also practicing telehealth. A broad definition is the application of health care services across space, time, social, and cultural barriers. Telehealth ideally involves changes both in technology and the health care environments where it is deployed (Fig. 14-1).

Telemedicine encompasses a range of specific medical activities including teleconsulting among clinicians, specialty telemedicine applications, tele-homecare, remote diagnosis, and remote surgery. Some of the specialty areas in which telemedicine has been employed include emergency medicine, cardiology, dermatology, ophthalmology, neurology, gastroenterology, rehabilitation, and critical care medicine.

Telemedicine and telehealth are associated with a variety of unique issues that have prompted legal scrutiny and legislative changes. One well-publicized example is the development of online pharmacies. In order to bypass ordinary constraints, consumers and providers have collaborated to form a marketplace for drugs to treat impotence, hair loss, and allergies. For example, "Internet doctors" maintain websites indicating that they "treat" erectile dysfunction. Interested patients describe their symptoms on a form, pay a fee, and are issued a prescription without ever having seen the physician. One company ran ads for physicians who would be willing to conduct "fully automated online medical reviews" in return for stipends of up to $10K per month. An orthopedist "reviewed" these forms and authorized sildanefil prescriptions in return for a stipend. It is hard to draw a clear line between this seemingly problematic interaction and legitimate tele-homecare, where a patient enters into a dialogue with an online physician to ask appropriate health care questions and receive care.

Another area with legal ramifications pertains to state licensure and malpractice in telemedicine. Traditionally medicine is practiced with both the patient and the clinician in the same place at the same time. Telemedicine permits separations in time and location. A clinician with a license in one state may interact with a patient in a different state during a virtual visit. A consultant in one state may collaborate with a clinician in another state or country during the care of a patient. For example, radiologists from the United States and Australia have taken advantage of the 12-hour difference between the two locations to facilitate 24-hour film reading (Fig. 14-2).

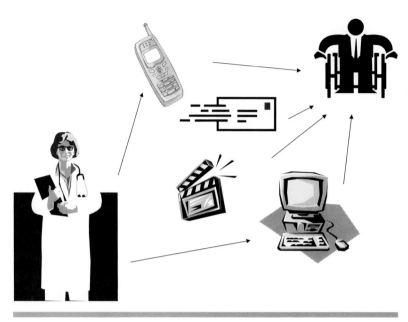

Figure 14-1
Telehealth is the delivery of healthcare over a distance using a variety of media.

Many of the legal, ethical, and reimbursement issues pertaining to telehealth and telemedicine have not been worked out. Inevitably, technological changes occur more rapidly than the responses to them.

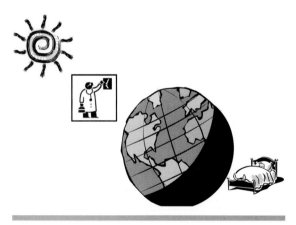

Figure 14-2
Radiologists in the United States read x-rays for Australian patients who are 12 hours out of synch, permitting Aussie radiologists to sleep.

History of Telemedicine

Key Points

■ Telemedicine dates back to the early 1900s and has used technologies including the radio, telephone, and videophone prior to today's use of the Internet.

■ Audio and video conferencing are two applications of two-way interactive telemedicine.

■ "Store and forward" telemedicine is exemplified by applications like teleradiology or telepathology, where data is acquired in one location at one time and can be viewed elsewhere at another time.

■ Teleimmersion and telepresence are next-generation tools for telemedicine.

Telemedicine is often thought of as a brand new idea. In fact, the concept of using telecommunications in the healthcare industry goes back to the early 1900s. There were early attempts using radio telecardiology (in the 1910s), telephone-mediated telestethoscopy (in the 1920s), and radiology image transfer and videophone experiments (in the early 1950s) (Fig. 14-3). The first generation of telemedicine using video conferencing began in the late 1950s with Dr. Cecil Wittson's microwave-mediated rural telepsychiatry program in Omaha, Nebraska, and with Dr. Albert Jutras' cable-mediated teleradiology program in Montreal.

The development of the Internet, widespread deployment of personal computers, emergence of a variety of standards, and greater confidence in these technologies by both the public and clinicians have facilitated the recent growth in telemedicine.

Some of the new technologies that are useful and appropriate for telemedicine-based healthcare are networking of various types including the Internet, satellite television, video conferencing, audio conferencing, and combinations of the foregoing technologies. Interactive multimedia is relatively mature and can be used to separate the development of a curriculum or evaluation tool from its deployment: for example, a medical self-assessment tool can be developed, burned onto a digital disk, and mass-mailed to subscribers. These techniques will seem primitive in the very near future, however.

Another way of classifying telemedicine technologies is to divide them into store and forward (i.e., unlinked in time) applications versus two-way interactive (i.e., real-time) applications. Typical examples of the former are teleradiology and tele-pathology, wherein images are acquired at one location, stored, and then forwarded to another for analysis or interpretation. Two-way interactions are used for consultation wherein a specialist is typically at one end of the link and a patient at another (Figs. 14-4 and 14-5).

New technologies that are currently under development include teleimmersion and telepresence. Teleimmersion combines components of video conferencing and virtual reality, permitting geographically dispersed people to collaborate in a shared virtual space, using shared resources (i.e., computer applications and multimedia). Telepresence refers to a human/machine system in which the human has visual and body-operated actuators and sensors permitting them to "see," "feel," and "move" (perhaps even "smell" and "taste") objects in a remote environment (Fig. 14-6). Three components are needed for this kind of interaction: the local or home user/machine technology, the communications link between the two, and the remote user/machine technology. While this concept is relevant to work in hostile environments (i.e., underwater, space, military settings), education, advertising, and entertainment, the most well-described medical application is remote, robotic surgery. In fact, a demonstration was done in 2001 where a surgeon in New York performed a laparoscopic cholecystectomy on a patient in France using robotic instruments.

Current Applications

Key Points

- Current telemedicine can be loosely divided into health services delivery, education and training, health administration, and telemedicine research.

- Health care delivery applications encompass applications within the acute healthcare setting, teleconsultation, home telehealth, and remote acute care.

- Best-practice approaches are readily applied using telemedicine health care delivery, which extends both the "reach" of individual clinicians as well as their approach to care.

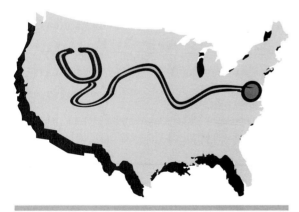

Figure 14-3
Telestethoscopy was one of the original telemedicine applications, wherein physicians auscultated remote patients.

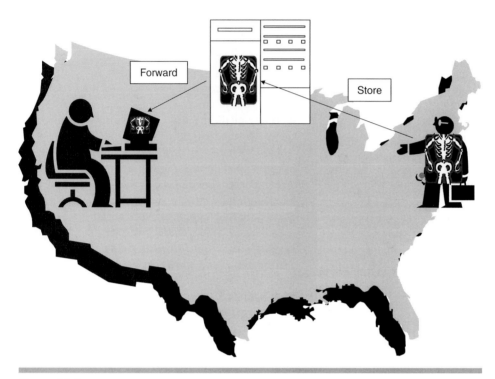

Figure 14-4
Store and forward is used for images such as x-rays or pathology slides.

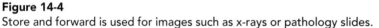

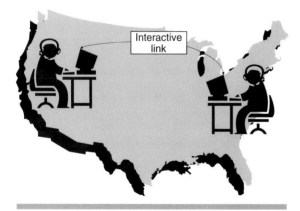

Figure 14-5
Two-way interactive communications uses media such as the Internet, phone system, or satellites.

The range of applications that currently fall under the aegis of telemedicine include four broad categories: health services, education and training, health administration, and research.

Health Services

Health services applications are varied and evolving daily. A brief description of several applications follows. Teleradiology is usually a store and forward application in which an image is acquired, either directly onto digital media or scanned into a file, and then sent on to a consultant to be read. Telepathology can be handled as a store and forward application; or a slide can be mounted on a remote microscope equipped with controls that allow the pathologist to manipulate the controls and thereby move the slide, change resolution, or focus. Teleintensive care allows a team of intensivists to monitor the vital signs, labs, and patient care

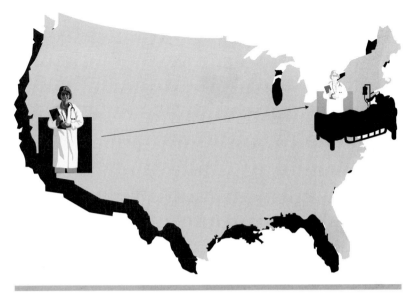

Figure 14-6
Telepresence refers to the ability to be "virtually" present in a patient care setting.

environment (using an audio and video link) of patients in multiple ICUs simultaneously (Fig. 14-7). This technology relies on real-time audio and video links from the remote location to the ICUs. Telepsychiatry also links a patient and clinician over a real-time interactive television link (as does tele-learning).

Wireless links can be used to transmit physiologic information from ambulances to destination emergency rooms, allowing the clinicians there to prepare adequately. Teleultrasound allows radiologists or obstetricians to examine remote patients by ultrasound.

Home telehealth is a growing model that allows clinicians to visit patients virtually, which is both cost-effective and convenient for the patient. Special tools have been designed for home- and clinic-based examinations such as networked manometers, glucometers, otoscopes, and stethoscopes.

The clinician can use data acquired from these devices and track trends of interest such as blood glucose values or blood pressure. The fact that these readings are acquired continuously and therefore are more representative of real life, makes them of

greater value than a fasting glucose on the day of an office visit or office blood pressure that might be affected by "white coat hypertension." Home telehealth permits the clinician and patient to establish daily, bidirectional communication (Fig. 14-8). Clinical information can be sent in either direction. A patient's health care patterns can be tracked over time and analyzed for deviations that might indicate a problem before it becomes acute. This proactive approach to care represents an attractive alternative to what is currently more of a crisis-management health care system.

Telemedicine applications have shown success in a variety of settings around the world. This technology has been used in rural settings, jails, and schools (i.e., school nurse) to extend the reach of clinicians. This enhances the care in underserved areas and eliminates the inconvenience to rural patients who might otherwise need to travel some distance to see a clinician. The cost and safety issues associated with the transportation of inmates from a correctional facility to a clinical site are minimized when the clinician handles most health care issues using a telemedicine link. The military and

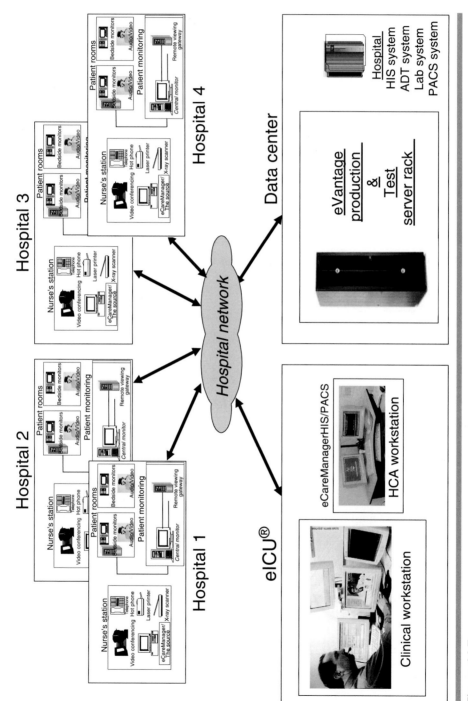

Figure 14-7
Teleintensive care architecture (courtesy of VISICU, Inc.).

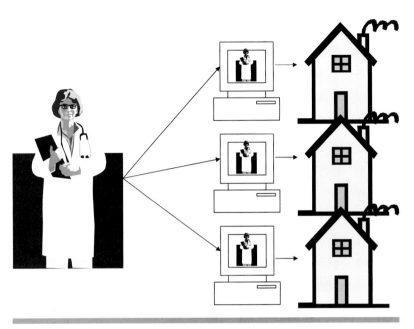

Figure 14-8
A clinician can make "virtual home calls" using telemedicine applications for the chronically ill.

travel industries are also ideal for telemedicine applications in which the clinician can evaluate a soldier or traveler rapidly when the time and location of illness are unpredictable.

Education and Training

The term telemedicine also encompasses "distance learning," where practitioners can be educated about specific topics or procedures using communications links. This approach is ideal for continuing education requirements as well as maximizing access to scarce educational resources (Fig. 14-9).

Health Administration

One of the "sales" points a telemedicine provider could make to potential client hospitals is access to its clinical guidelines, protocols, and pathways. As an example, the ICU telemedicine provider might give the client hospital access to a bundle of internally developed ICU practices such as deep vein thrombosis prevention, ventilator associated pneumonia prevention, and stress ulcer prophylaxis. Legal questions arise as to the potential liability of

the provider hospital for issues relating to patient care at the client hospital implementing those practices. Conversely, a client hospital may be liable for blindly following poorly conceived guidelines or for failing to consistently follow guidelines.

Telemedicine Research

While the potential benefits of telemedicine in patient care are obvious, little research has been done to "prove" that those benefits are real or realizable. Governments are funding demonstration projects in a number of fields to determine which applications of telemedicine are likely to show the greatest benefit to which patient populations.

■ Barriers

Key Points

- There are a variety of impediments to the rapid dissemination of telemedicine including the lack of reimbursement models, licensure, malpractice, credentialing, and antitrust legislation.

- Insurers are gradually developing approaches to reimbursement for telehealth.

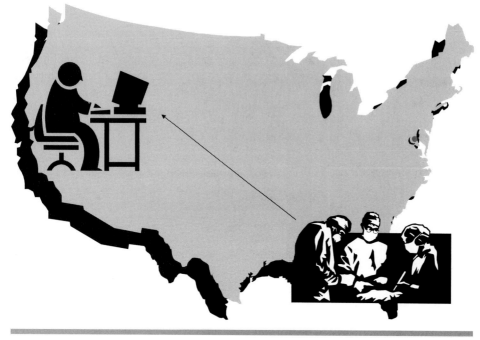

Figure 14-9
Telemedicine is ideally suited for continuing education and distance learning.

■ There are a variety of potential models relating to licensure for delivery of telehealth across state lines, none of which are universally accepted.

■ Malpractice liability for the delivery of telehealth is unclear and precedents are lacking.

■ It is unclear how antitrust legislation applies to relationships among providers using a telehealth network.

Telemedicine represents a major shift in focus for reimbursement entities such as Medicare, Medicaid, and private payers. One of the essential elements to most reimbursable medical encounters is the presence of the clinician at the point of care. Insurers have been reluctant to pay for telemedical care fearing that payment codes for care of this sort may be abused and cause an upswing in already burgeoning medical costs. Some progress has been made as demonstration projects have been shown to be successful and cost-effective.

Reimbursement

Medicare legislation enacted in 2000 was designed to improve Medicare reimbursement in regards to eligibility criteria, coverage, conditions of payment, and methods of payment. The geographic areas eligible for telemedicine reimbursement include nonmetropolitan counties and a variety of demonstration sites. The services that can be billed include telemedical consultation, office visits, psychotherapy, and pharmacologic management (i.e., insulin adjustment) delivered via a telecommunications link. Coverage includes both interactive television and "store and forward" applications in certain locations. The payment to the remote clinician is equivalent to what it would have been were the visit actual rather than virtual.

Medicare has been a leader in developing reimbursement strategies for telemedical care. Other payers are beginning to follow suit as the potential benefits to underserved patient populations are better understood. Other barriers remain, however including issues pertaining to licensure and malpractice.

Licensure

Many states prohibit the practice of medicine by out-of-state clinicians, and the site of care has traditionally been at the location of the patient (Fig. 14-10). The regulation of licensure is the purview of each state, and the issues that arise relating to state-by-state licensure and telemedicine are manifold. The licensure process is complicated and costly as the state attempts to ensure the competence and quality of the physicians that practice within its borders. The acquisition and maintenance of a state license is time consuming and costly for the practitioner. Some states require appearances before a board; some require the passage of a test. Maintenance of multiple licenses is challenging for a practitioner and therefore an impediment to the practice of telemedicine outside of a given state.

The states have varied models relating to the provision of telemedical care, if they specify them at all. Some of the potential approaches include special telemedicine licensure, reciprocal agreements between or among states, limited licensure, registration, blanket permission for consultations, and prohibition of a primary care relationship to a patient without full licensure (Table 14-1). The Federation of State Medical Boards has outlined a model act in which the telemedical practitioner could practice cybermedicine within a state after having obtained a limited license in each state.

Some of the recommended guidelines relate to evaluation, documentation, treatment standards,

Table 14-1 Licensure alternatives

Telemedicine license

Reciprocal agreement between/among states

Full license requirement

Limited license

Permission for telemedicine consultation only

National cyber license with limited state license

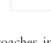

Figure 14-10
There are licensure barriers relating to the practice of telemedicine across state lines.

electronic communication, informed consent, medical records, and compliance with state and federal law. For example, the federation states that the issuance of a prescription (i.e., sildenafil) based on information acquired from a web-based form is inappropriate. Electronic communications should be secure, based on existing technologies, and records of those communications should be stored in the patient's medical record. Informed consent documents should address limitations due to technical failures such as the loss of electronic data due to network issues. Physicians who practice through Internet web sites are engaged in the practice of medicine and should be held to applicable standards. These are but a few, representative recommendations from the federation.

Malpractice

Rapidly escalating malpractice coverage costs for routine care have increased the visibility of this issue to the point that it was a debate point in the recent presidential campaign. Physicians have retired or refused to practice in many states. The American Medical Association has identified states that are facing medical liability crises. With this backdrop, telemedicine is maturing and forcing the consideration of questions such as who is liable in care involving both a home and remote physician, to whom do the risks associated with telemedicine equipment failures fall, and who is responsible for obtaining informed consent prior to remote, robotic surgery.

Malpractice issues arise in the provision of telemedicine both for the individual clinician and for the components of network. Take the case of a health system that provides critical care telemedicine services to a nonaffiliated hospital. The health system employs the critical care nurses and provides practice protocols. The complicated interrelationships inherent in the delivery of care in this scenario, and the absence of legal precedents make it difficult to say who would be liable should a problem arise with a patient at the client hospital.

Another example relates to the relationship between a physician and patients over an Internet link. The physician cannot see, touch, or hear the patient, so the question arises as to whether it is a patient-physician relationship in the formal sense. To what extent are the communications and recommendations subject to laws regarding traditional medical interactions?

Credentialing

State law and accreditation organizations require hospitals to credential providers and to make sure that providers are competent in their areas of practice. Different hospitals, even within a network, can have different proficiency standards. Telemedicine is a new area and every hospital engaging in this practice, either as a provider or recipient, will have to draft medical bylaws changes to reflect the practice of telemedicine. One relevant question relates to whether there should be separate standards for "virtual" practice. Should remote (i.e., telemedicine consultant) physicians be admitted to the medical staff to practice in the hospital? If so, should telemedicine consultants be subjected to the same scrutinies as other medical staff members and to what degree are they subject to the same sanctions?

Antikickback and antitrust issues

One logical consequence of the development of a telemedicine relationship between hospitals is new patient referral patterns. Medicare prohibits arrangements where one purpose is to offer, solicit, or pay anything of value in return for patient referrals for treatment or services paid for by Medicare, Medicaid, or state program. This raises questions pertaining to relationships wherein a telemedicine provider subsidizes or gives equipment to a client hospital and that hospital refers patients back to the provider. For example, if equipment was given to the ICU in a local hospital to facilitate monitoring of patients in the unit by a tertiary ICU telemedicine provider, would it be a violation to send critically ill patients to the tertiary ICU? Similar questions arise as to antitrust and anticompetitive practices in network webs.

Conclusion

Telemedicine will unquestionably change the way that medicine is practiced in many fundamental ways. It is equally certain that the speed of technological change will outstrip that of regulatory, reimbursement, and legislative change.

Suggested Readings

Norris AC. *Essentials of Telemedicine and Telecare*. New York: John Wiley & Sons, 2002.

Darkins AW, Cary MA. *Telemedicine and Telehealth: Principles, Policies, Performance and Pitfalls*. Springer, 2000.

15 HIPAA

Introduction and History

Key Points

- The Healthcare Insurance Portability and Accountability Act (HIPAA) legislation as we know it represents the marriage of two very different legislative efforts.

- The portability component was intended to prevent workers from losing health coverage when they transitioned between jobs.

- Accountability relates to the increasing vulnerability of health information in the electronic age and the responsibility health care workers have to protect it.

The HIPAA act of 1996 was designed to protect workers from losing their ability to be covered by health insurance (portability) on leaving a job, and to protect the integrity, confidentiality, and availability of electronic health information (accountability). Because of its complexity, resistance, and the difficulty and cost of implementation, several delays took place prior to its final implementation which is not surprising given the fact that the initial roots of the act go back several decades.

In 1975, a group of health care providers met with payers to discuss the creation of a standard hospital claim form. This was obviously well before the beginning of the personal computer era and the Internet; but the committee that resulted, the National Uniform Billing Committee, created a form called the UB-82 claim form which became an industry standard.

While standardization was the initial goal, other drivers began to emerge for health care efficiency as costs began to escalate in the latter part of the

1980s. In the early 1990s, the first Bush administration called together a group of industry leaders to address approaches to the reduction of health care costs. One of the conclusions of the group was that electronic data interchange should lead to the elimination of paper claims submission. Interestingly, an American Hospital Association study done in 1988 indicate that more than 60% of the insurance claims were submitted electronically at that point, using the UB-82 form.

The Workgroup for Electronic Data Interchange (WEDI) resulted from the Bush era initiative and, after a good deal of study, recommended that federal legislation should be enacted describing consistent national standards for electronic data interchange. These recommendations were included in the Clinton health plan, which failed to pass Congress; however, they ultimately became a part of the House version of the HIPAA legislation passed in 1996.

The HIPAA law is more commonly thought of as being the product of efforts by Senators Edward Kennedy and Nancy Kassebaum, who created legislation designed to ensure the portability of health insurance. The need for laws of this sort emerged, again due to escalating health care costs, as health insurers began to refuse coverage to vulnerable parties such as those with preexisting conditions, pregnancy, or transitions between jobs.

The electronic data interchange and health care portability aspects of the HIPAA legislation were married when the former was attached to the latter during its passage through Congress (Table 15-1), largely due to the efforts of Representative David Hobson. The final bill had two major sections. The first, Title I, addresses Health Care Access,

Table 15-1 Outline of HIPAA*

Title I: Health care access, portability, and renewability	
Access	Guarantees access to health insurance
Portability	Guarantees portability of health insurance between jobs
Renewability	Guarantees renewability of health insurance
Title II: Preventing fraud and abuse: administrative simplification	
Fraud and abuse programs and sanctions	Program to address health care fraud
Administrative simplification	Privacy, electronic data interchange and security provisions
Duplication of Medicare plans	Relates to Medicare coverage in certain instances
Title III: Tax-related health provisions	
Title IV: Application and enforcement of group health plan requirements	
Title V: Revenue offsets	

*Privacy, electronic data interchange, and security are what most people think of as HIPAA because they have had the most direct impact on patient care.

Portability, and Renewability. Its first objective is guarantee health insurance coverage to all employees and families (access). The second focus of Title I is health insurance portability (five aspects).

Title II is of greater relevance to the topic of this book: Preventing Health Care Fraud and Abuse, Administrative Simplification; Medical Liability Reform. The fraud and abuse section established a Fraud and Abuse Control System and lies outside of the scope of this chapter. The Administrative Simplification section deals both with electronic data interchange and data security.

This section also led to the development of standards for privacy of individually identifiable health information by the Department of Health and Human Services. The addition of security and privacy language to the HIPAA bill was prompted by increased public awareness of the vulnerability of medical data. For example, tennis star Arthur Ashe declared the fact that he had AIDS in large part due to the fact that he was convinced that a national newspaper was about to publish that information without his permission.

HIPAA Components

Key Points

- HIPAA has three aspects that relate to the computerization of medical information and patient's rights
- Privacy
- Code sets
- Security
- Privacy refers to the requirement for health care deliverers to obtain consent from patients as to the management of their protected health information (PHI).
- Code sets refers to the tags and labels used in the identification of patient-specific data, including disease definitions, billing codes, and patient identifiers.
- Security covers the administrative, physical, and technical safeguards used to protect patient data.

The components of HIPAA that relate to the development of electronic data, security, and privacy standards have had major implications for the health care industry and focused attention on the implications of computerization of medical information as they relate to patient' rights. There are three key aspects of HIPAA that relate to computerization: privacy, code sets and security. The latter is further broken down into four parts: administrative procedures, physical safeguards, technical security services (which refers to the passage of data across an intranet contained within a healthcare entity), and technical security mechanisms (covering data as it transitions across a nonprivate network).

Privacy

The privacy aspect of HIPAA covers health plans, health care clearinghouses, and health care providers who deal in electronic billing and funds transfers. Additionally, this part of the legislation defines the term PHI. It also provides the patient with greater access to and control of their medical record and data (Fig. 15-1).

HIPAA requires a covered entity (health care provider) to obtain prospective approval from a patient prior to sharing PHI with organizations such as insurance companies, billing companies, physicians to whom a patient might be referred, or other covered entities.

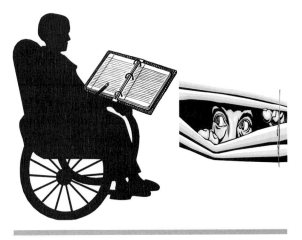

Figure 15-1
The HIPAA privacy requirement gives the patient access to and control of their medical data and its accessibility to others.

This portion of HIPAA evoked substantial resistance from the healthcare community, which supported the privacy concept but had major objections to the initial implementation rules. There was concern that many provisions of the initial version of the legislation could prevent timely patient care in the event of an emergency. They objected that it was inappropriate to delay treatment in an emergency situation, for example, while the patient pored through and signed off on lengthy privacy forms.

The initial rule was modified under the second Bush administration to eliminate a requirement to obtain patient consent for the use of their PHI for routine healthcare delivery purposes. The final privacy rule was published in 2002 and had strengthened provisions for patient notification of privacy rights and barriers to the use of patient information for marketing purposes.

Electronic Data Interchange

HIPAA describes medical code sets and identifiers. The former include any sets of codes used for encoding medical data elements, such as tables of terms, medical concepts, medical diagnosis codes, procedures codes, and medications. Some common examples of code sets include the International Classification of Diseases (ICD) from the World Health Organization and the Current Procedural Terminology (CPT).

There are many identifiers used in electronic medical data interchange. They include the National Provider ID, which is used to uniquely identify healthcare providers. The National Employer ID is used to identify employers and other health care benefits sponsors who use EDI to enroll members in health care plans or pay benefits premiums. Health plan IDs are used to identify health plans such as Medicare contractors, Medicaid programs, and other insurers.

The concept of a National Patient ID was raised and never enacted due a variety of concerns about the privacy implications of such a number. Most of the concerns center on the potential for linkage of such a number to other sensitive data, such as financial information, employment records, and so on. For example, it is already clear that, given a few identifiers it is easy to "steal" an individual's electronic identity. The social security number is an example of a number that is in widespread use and one with major inherent privacy implications. While it is reasonable to expect that a unique number will eventually come into use as part of a universal patient record (Chap. 9), it is not yet clear what form that number will take and what protections will be put in place for its use (Fig. 15-2).

In addition to the identifiers described above, standards have been described for a variety of forms analogous to the progenitor UB-82 claim. These include forms relating to enrollment, encounters, claims, benefits, referrals, and injury reports.

Security

Without security provisions, much of the other components of the legislation would be unenforceable. The security rules cover policies, procedures, physical safeguards, and technical aspects of the management of PHI.

The general provision of the rule is designed to ensure the confidentiality, integrity, and availability of electronic PHI that a covered entity creates, receives, maintains, or transmits. It also requires the covered entity (i.e. hospital, nursing home, or doctor's office) to take action to protect against any reasonably anticipated threats to the security or integrity of PHI as well as impermissible use or disclosure of that information. The covered entity is responsible for ensuring the compliance of the workforce it employs.

Some of the key aspects of the administrative rules of HIPAA relate to risk analysis, risk management, sanctions, and information systems activity review. There are rules relating to the management of the employed workforce, such as supervision, clearance, and termination procedures. An example of a potential risk would be the termination of an employee and the failure to concurrently remove access to PHI. The terminated employee might have access to a patient's data while no longer covered by the covered entity's policies and sanctions. There are also rules addressing employee access authorization and modification.

Another evolving risk addressed by this section relates to security reminders and preventative efforts pertaining to malicious software such as viruses and worms. Computer systems should be equipped with updated antiviral software, for example, to prevent critical medical systems from attacks that might have harmful effects on patient care. Password management and the monitoring of attempts to log on to a system are designed to thwart hackers who might attempt to gain access to PHI for prurient or malicious reasons (Fig. 15-3).

The administrative rules require covered entities to attempt to identify and respond to suspected or known security incidents (such as an attempt to hack into a protected data base) as well as to document them. The components of a disaster plan relate to data back-up both within the system as well as at redundant off-site, "disaster-resistant" locations. In addition, the entity is required to have a disaster recovery plan and emergency mode operation plan (in the event of an interruption of power or network access) (Fig. 15-4).

Physical Safeguards The physical security of medical data is equal in importance to the electronic

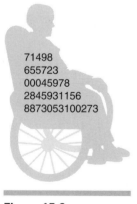

71498
655723
00045978
2845931156
8873053100273

Figure 15-2
HIPAA contemplates the creation of a universal patient identification number, which has significant privacy implications.

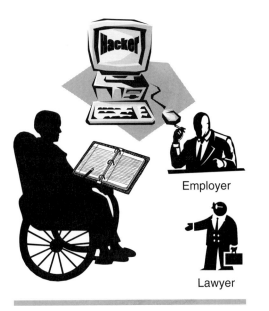

Figure 15-3
There are a variety of potential threats to electronic medical data with different motivations and capabilities.

safeguards. HIPAA has rules describing facility access controls and validation procedures for staff and visitors to a health care facility as well the maintenance of computer hardware.

Computer terminals are points of vulnerability in the management of PHI. Computers that are in public locations are at potential risk. The physical location and visibility of computer screens should be evaluated to ensure that unauthorized viewing is not possible (Fig. 15-5). For example, a computer screen used for documentation in an EHR should not be placed so that it can be read by a hospital visitor. Printers and fax machines used to create documents containing PHI should be in secure locations. Locks, keys, and other devices should be used to control access to locations containing computer systems.

Finally, both paper and electronic media containing PHI should be subject to specific controls to prevent unauthorized access. Paper records should be shredded. Reusable electronic media should be erased prior to reuse in unprotected locations. For example, it is relatively easy to recover information from a computer disk even after a file has been "deleted," and there is an entire field of forensic computer science devoted to the extraction of usable data from disks that have been erased and/or physically damaged.

The typical approach to deletion of a file is to "delete" it or drag it to the "Trashcan" or "Recycle Bin" depending on the operating system. Many

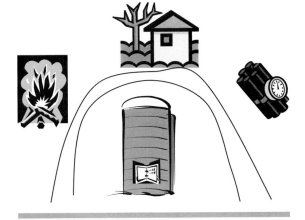

Figure 15-4
Copies of electronic medical data should be stored in off-site, disaster-resistant storage facilities.

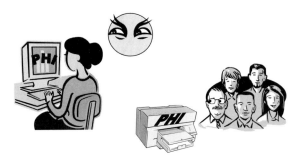

Figure 15-5
Physical safeguards should be in place to prevent inappropriate viewing of protected health information.

users think that the file is finally deleted after the bin or can is "emptied." This second step merely erases the file pointers to the data, leaving the data intact on the disk until it is overwritten by new data. It may be a while before new data completely overwrites an old file. Even after this point, special software can be used to recover some overwritten data, because new data do not necessarily fall exactly on top of old data—there may be an offset of a new bit relative to the old one on a magnetic disk platter. It is easy to imagine that computers that are discarded or resold after use in a medical facility may have easily recoverable PHI, much as dumpsters containing discarded paper records are vulnerable.

Technical Safeguards Technical security services and mechanisms refer to the management of PHI stored on an intranet. HIPAA indicates that PHI stored within an intranet must be securely stored and that access to it must be strictly regulated. This rule includes issues such as logging onto the network (authorization which is typically the user's computer identification), authentication (usually the password).

The combination of user ID and password will almost certainly be supplanted or augmented by new technologies such as biometric identifiers in the near future. An example of a biometric marker that is readily acquired and for which the technology is maturing is fingerprints. Touchpad fingerprint acquisition and authentication tools can be used to ensure that the individual logging on to a system is who they say they are, and can be used in addition to existing security measures (Fig. 15-6).

Once a user is authenticated, HIPAA mandates that some form of audit trail is maintained as the user interacts with the computer system. The manifest of each interaction with the system must be kept for a period of time, and can be retroactively analyzed. It is likely that health care systems will create multitiered access at some point in the future. For example, there are many reasons to limit access to HIV status or psychiatric PHI to a limited set of clinicians by creating a specific tier for access to that data.

HIPAA requires the development of formalized policies for the management of forgotten or suspect

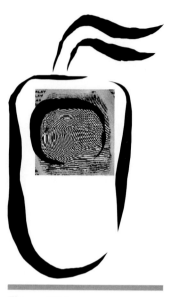

Figure 15-6
Biometric fingerprint identification, using a biometric mouse for example, can be used to ensure accurate authentication during the use of PHI.

(i.e., possibly "stolen") passwords, the use of email, and access to workstations. Some institutions have chosen to forbid the use of laptop computers on an intranet to prevent easy downloading and physical removal of PHI from a site. Additional rules require the creation of policies designed to prevent improper alteration or destruction of PHI. This "data integrity" standard is designed to prevent malicious or inadvertent mismanagement of electronic PHI.

In addition to the maintenance of data that is stored, HIPAA has rules relating to data that is "in motion," i.e. being transmitted over a network such as the Internet, a virtual private network (VPN), or a private, "leased" line. HIPAA originally mandated encryption of such data, but now only recommends consideration of encryption. The primary reason for this retrenchment is the potential cost to smaller covered entities and the fact that simple, interoperable email solutions are not yet readily available. Data transmitted across a VPN is encrypted by definition, but transmission of unencrypted PHI across the Internet is still possible under existing HIPAA regulations (Fig. 15-7).

Business Associates

The nature of business in today's health care environment is that many parties are intertwined in the management of PHI, such as providers, payers, contractors, and so on. For example, a covered entity may license software, such as an electronic health record, from a software vendor. The vendor is likely to require some form of access to the computer systems on which the software is installed and the databases containing PHI that are created by that software. The vendor's employees are not directly bound by the rules and policies of the covered entity.

HIPAA requires a business associate agreement for relationships where the vendor creates, maintains, receives, or transmits PHI on behalf of the covered entity. This rule requires the vendor to implement the same kind of safeguards that the entity does to ensure the protection of PHI on behalf of the entity. It requires the vendor to report security breaches to the entity. It also mandates the inclusion of language in the contract authorizing termination of the relationship if the vendor violates the rules pertaining to the protection of PHI.

Conclusion

The HIPAA legislation has a fascinating history and in many ways is analogous to an animal designed by a committee or the elephant as perceived by the three blind men. In spite of this, the legislation addresses a number of important issues essential to patient care in an era of computerized medicine. New violations of general privacy rights are reported daily in the news, including identity theft, systematic theft of information from data vendors, and inappropriate release of sensitive medical data. For example, three major data vendors have reported the theft of names, addresses, drivers' licenses, social security numbers, and medical information within recent months. Similarly, a public health official recently inadvertently appended a

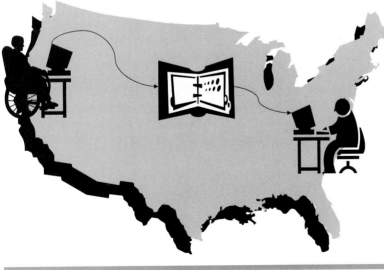

Figure 15-7
"Data in motion" refers to PHI as it moves across media such as phone lines, networks, or satellites.

list of HIV positive residents to a general email distribution.

As originally constructed, HIPAA provided a series of rigid rules that amounted to an unfunded mandate, and one which would have essentially been impossible to realize for small covered entities such as private physicians' practices. While the law was passed in 1996, it has undergone staged implementation during which it was substantially revised after periods of public comment and retooling. Some of the original mandates, such as the creation of a national, unique patient identifier were eliminated. Others were changed significantly, such as the requirement for patient preauthorization prior to the acquisition of PHI during the process of patient care.

In its current version, the HIPAA legislation represents a relatively flexible set of rules that anticipate changes in technology and yet are achievable today. HIPAA very quickly became a watchword in the health care industry and has resulted in dramatic and rapid changes in the way paper, electronic, and even verbal PHI is thought of and managed.

Suggested Readings

Beaver K, Herold R. *The Practical Guide to HIPAA Privacy and Security Compliance.* Auerbach Publications CRC Press LLC, Boca Raton, Florida, 2003.

Dinkins C, Gilbreath A. *HIPAA in Daily Practice.* Kerlak Enterprises Kerlak Publications, Memphis, Tennessee, 2003.

Pabrai UOA. *Getting Started with HIPAA.* Muska & Lipman/Premier-Trade, Premier Press, Boston, Massachusetts, 2003.

Multimedia in Medicine

Introduction

Key Points

- Digital records of sound, still, and moving images are increasingly prevalent in medical care.
- Medical records are being digitized.
- The efficient storage and transmission of digital information depends on digital compression.
- The use of digital formats permits the application of the same digital signal enhancement techniques that have been depicted in forensically oriented television and movies.

Still and moving digital images are increasingly becoming a part of the medical record, which will no doubt ultimately become a mixed multimedia virtual document encompassing many different types of information. This could conceivably include audio or video recordings of doctor-patient interactions, perhaps even records of auscultation and or the physical examination of a patient using haptic technology (Fig. 16-1).

Records of this kind will be "bulky" when first acquired and they will probably undergo some degree of compression prior to storage and/or transmission. Additionally, because they are digital, multimedia files are susceptible to computerized techniques for enhancement of the signal of interest (i.e., sound, picture) (Fig. 16-2).

This chapter provides a brief introduction to the concepts and implications of data compression, transmission and manipulation, and their application in a medical setting, and will focus primarily on still images and video, although the same principles are applicable to sound as well.

Digital Recording Basics

Key Points

- The same data, be it sound or image, can be stored in a variety of ways with significantly different degrees of efficiency, portability, and integrity depending on what format is used.
- A large variety of storage formats have been developed, and they differ in their intent—some are designed for faithful (lossless) reproduction of data others for efficient storage (lossy).
- Many data storage formats have a large amount of "empty space" such as the white are on a piece of newspaper.
- Compression is used in all of our communications (i.e., telephony) and usually with no significant impact on our comprehension.

Information can be stored in many ways, some of which are inherently inefficient relative to others. For example, an interval of sound can be stored on a wire, a polyvinyl chloride platter, or CD. Similarly, a document can be stored as a printed piece of paper or a sequence of letters and formatting codes used by a word processing program to arrange the letters. The same letter can also be stored as a picture image, as a digital camera, copier or fax machine would record it. The proprietary Adobe "pdf" format offers yet another method of storing the same document. Depending on which format is used, the same information can take up very different amounts of storage space (Fig. 16-3).

Document storage is obviously a major issue as medical records are moved from paper and microfiche to online repositories. Compression is essential for the efficient storage and transmission of

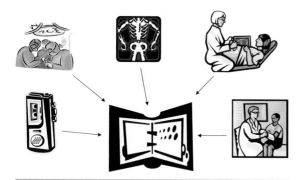

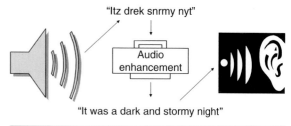

"Itz drek snrmy nyt"

"It was a dark and stormy night"

Figure 16-2
Computers can be used to enhance signals of interest in audio and visual data.

Figure 16-1
A variety of digital information including still images, audio files, video data, and perhaps even recordings of examinations will become part of the electronic medical record of the future.

images and videos. Internet telephony and digital dictation are two examples of digital sounds that are beginning to be used for communication in hospitals.

Data compression sounds like a formidable topic, but it is fundamental to many computer-based applications and figures prominently in medical applications. Data compression, in computer science, is defined as the process of encoding an original information file using fewer bits than were used to store the original image.

One of the most familiar and oldest methods of compression is known as the "zip" format. The zip

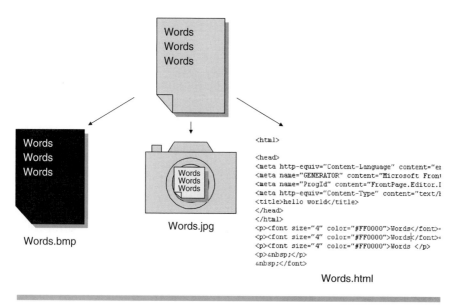

Figure 16-3
The exact same document can be stored in a variety of different formats, including bit mapped (left), photographic (center), and hypertext (right), with very different storage implications.

format was originally developed as one of several methods to enhance the speed and efficiency with which data was downloaded from dial-up "bulletin-boards." Bulletin-boards predate the Internet and were used as common repositories for the storage of computer files such as program updates, pictures, "freeware," and "shareware."

There are a large variety of other compression formats in common use. Some of the more familiar ones include the "gif" (graphics interchange format) and "jpg" (joint photographics expert group) for pictures, the "wav" (WAVEform audio format, a Microsoft and IBM audio format) and "mp3" audio formats, and the "mpg" (moving picture experts group) and "avi" (audio-video interleave) formats (Tables 16-1 and 16-2).

One key to the use of any of these formats is that the sending (or saving) and receiving (or retrieving) software clients must employ the same compression algorithm. For example, if a sender encodes an email attachment using the zip format, the receiver must have a program capable of decoding the "zipped" file in order to read it. Note that the terms encoding and decoding here are analogous to compress and decompress. In fact, there are many similarities to the processes involved in compression and encryption.

Compression is possible because much of the information that we work with, be it static or moving pictures, or sound, is very redundant or inherently inconcise when it is represented in a "human-accessible" format. Consider the amount of white space on a typical page such as this. All

Table 16-2   Common audio and video formats

Extension	Developer	Use
Audio		
.mid	MIDI manufacturers	Synthesizers
.mp3	Open source	Internet and players
.ra/.ram	RealAudio	Streaming
.wav	Microsoft	Audio CD
Video		
.avi	Microsoft	General-purpose
.mov	Apple Quicktime	Best-quality
.mpg	Open source	General-purpose
.rm/.ram	RealVideo	Streaming
.swf	Macromedia	Web-pages
.wmv	Microsoft	General purpose

of the white space is faithfully represented in a picture of the page and yet it is all devoid of meaning (Fig. 16-4).

Compression is an important way of reducing the inefficiency of data representation and can reduce the use of expensive resources such as disk space. However, there is also a cost inherent in compression due to the computing power needed to compress the information. As memory storage costs decrease and computing power increases, many of these considerations have lost relevance. It is now practical, for example, to scan years of

Table 16-1   Common still image formats

Format	Loss	Compressed	Use
.bmp	Lossless	Rarely	Photographs/graphics
.gif	Lossless	Yes	Clipart/animated figures
.jpg	Lossy	Yes	Photographs
.png	Lossless	Yes	Alternative to .gif
.pdf	Lossless	No	Documents
.tiff	Lossless	No	Photographs, publishing

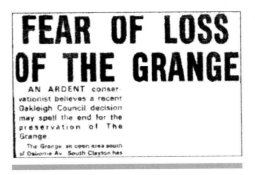

Figure 16-4
Typical storage formats have a large amount of wasted, data-less space.

medical records files into computers at a cost that is acceptable to hospitals.

One concept that is essential to an understanding of compression is "lossy" versus "lossless" algorithms (described in chapter). Lossy compression algorithms preserve some fraction of the original information (depending on the approach and the settings selected by the user), permitting more or less faithful reconstruction of the original file. Lossless approaches are completely reversible and permit complete reconstruction (Fig. 16-5).

Data compression is important for efficient storage, but is also critical for the transmission of information across communications networks. Much of the information we work with is compressed in some format. Pictures transmitted across the Internet are compressed. Communications hardware like modems, bridges, and routers use compression to increase the amount of data that can be transmitted over standard phone lines. Compression is used to compress voice telephone calls so that more calls can be placed on the same lines. Compression is also essential for video conferencing applications that run over data networks (Fig. 16-6).

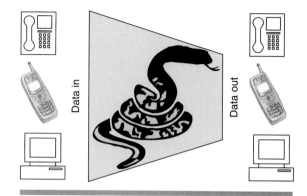

Figure 16-6
Much of the data we work with in our daily lives is compressed during the process of transmission from its source.

Digital signal enhancement is commonly thought of in conjunction with military or forensic applications, but the techniques that are used to enhance a satellite photograph of a military installation are equally applicable to the enhancement of a chest radiograph. The ability to alter a chest x-ray interactively can be of significant benefit to the radiologist (Fig. 16-7).

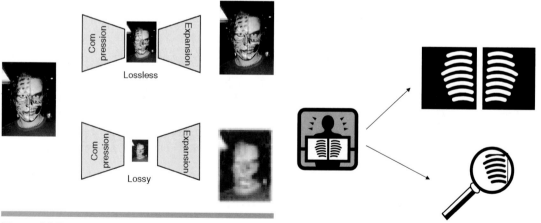

Figure 16-5
Lossless compression techniques retain all of the information to completely reconstruct the original whereas lossy techniques compress more effectively but lose information.

Figure 16-7
Digital image enhancement permits functions like digital zoom, contrast enhancement, black-white reversal, and so on.

Still Picture Formats and Compression

Key Points

- Many forms of medical image data are being converted to or captured directly as digital files.

- Some of the common image formats include "bmp," "gif," and "jpg" and they differ as to whether they are compressed or lossy.

- There are medial-legal ramifications to the way in which image data is stored.

- Image enhancement has replaced many older methods of managing low-quality images.

Issues pertaining to picture compression are increasingly relevant to physicians as more photographic information becomes computerized. Radiology images, endoscopy, or surgical pictures and pathology slides are examples of medical images that a clinician is likely to encounter online to an increasing degree.

A chest x-ray is a typical example of the kind of picture that a clinician might have occasion to view in the course of patient care. Historically, chest x-rays have been captured on film while more recently most images are captured on charge coupled devices (CCDs). Compared with CCDs, film x-rays require higher patient radiation doses, photographic development and are not reusable. They are higher resolution but not readily susceptible to image manipulation. CCD images are captured on reusable plates and can be immediately viewed on a computer after "exposure." The digital nature of the CCD data means that it can be manipulated in the same way that any other digital photographic image can, using software designed for that purpose. Another advantage of digital x-rays is the fact that they can both be stored on a primary radiology storage medium and compressed for transmission over or viewing on the Internet (Fig. 16-8).

There are a variety of common image formats as mentioned. The "bmp" format is both uncompressed and lossless, and files in that format therefore tend to be large. The "gif" format is frequently used on the Internet. It provides for efficient, albeit

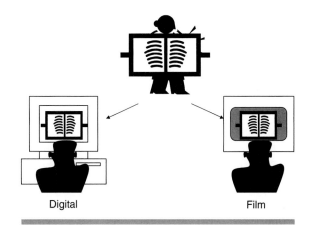

Figure 16-8
Digital x-rays are recorded in an electronically accessible format, whereas traditional x-rays are captured on photographic film.

lossy, compression. Unlike "jpg" compression it is very efficient at compressing images with expanses of flat or uniform colors (such as cartoon characters). However, GIF images eliminate a great deal of information about color gradations or shades of gray and because of the latter are not well suited to compression of radiographic data. JPG images are ideal for photographs or radiographs because JPG compression preserves most of the information about subtle gradation during the compression process. A file that is originally 4 megabytes in size, for example, can be compressed to a 50-kilobyte file with minimal image degradation.

Most chest radiographs are approximately 1 megabyte in size when originally acquired on a CCD plate, and can therefore be compressed to very small, efficiently handled files for transmission. One other photographic standard format is the TIFF (tagged image file format). This is used very commonly in graphic design and publication applications because it is well accepted and lossless. However, because TIFF files are uncompressed and therefore very large, they are unsuited to web-based image viewing. The best compression that lossless approaches are likely to achieve is on the order of 2–3:1, whereas JPG compression can do orders of magnitude better. A widely used alternative to JPG compression, called wavelet compression is used in the archiving of radiographic images and allows radiologists to determine the degree of compression used for specific films or applications.

One of the key considerations to any computer-based manipulation of medical information relates to its integrity during the manipulation, i.e., can the information/image be recreated for medico-legal review. A lossy compression technique is problematic in that the compressed x-ray is not an exactly faithful reproduction of the original (Fig. 16-9). There are risks associated with storing a compressed version of the original, in that the information has now been altered should a subsequent lawsuit arise. Similarly, if the radiologist's original reading is made on a compressed image, they could be faulted for having missed a lesion discovered subsequently on a later film. The question then arises as to whether the lesion was originally missed due to malpractice or lossy compression. Suffice it to say that there are a number of tradeoffs involved that are specific to the interpretation and archiving of x-rays, but that compression is essential for web-based image distribution.

In computer graphics, the process of improving the quality of a digitally stored image by manipulating it with software is called image enhancement. It is easy, for example, to change brightness and contrast, and digital x-rays are typically normalized for optimal interpretation eliminating the wide variability in brightness typical of film-based x-rays. Advanced image enhancement software also supports many tools and filters for altering images in various ways. Programs specialized for image enhancement are called image editors and many image management functions are built into today's PACS stations.

The traditional x-ray viewing paradigm has been transillumination of an x-ray. Films of varying contrast (due to differing penetration of the x-rays through the body part of interest to the film on the far side) were compared side-by-side. Bright spotlights and magnifying glasses were used as tools to assist in reading "dark" films or magnify an area of interest.

Bright lights have been replaced by tools allowing the viewer to control the black/white gradient. PACS software provides tools to zoom in on or magnify areas of an x-ray. Two techniques are used in these processes, pixel replication and interpolation. In either process, a subset of the original pixels is used to create a larger image; therefore, new pixels have to be created. With pixel replication, a single pixel is replicated with additional pixels of the same value, whereas with pixel interpolation, pixels of intermediate value are created and interpolated between the original pixels. Digital subtraction (black-white reversal) is useful for certain applications. A "stack" of two-dimensional images such as a CT scan series can be created and scanned through to permit simulation of three-dimensional viewing. Precise measurement tools (to measure the size of or distance between objects) are built into PACS software (Table 16-3).

There are a number of additional image enhancement technologies that are not in widespread use today that may enhance image analysis in the future, such as edge enhancement algorithms. Computer-aided diagnosis is likely to grow in importance in much the same way that computer-aided ECG analysis is now common.

Video Formats and Compression

Key Points

- In the same way that still images are being digitized and transmitted, medical video is increasingly prevalent.

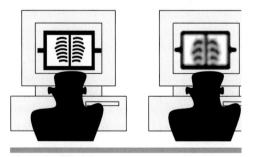

Figure 16-9
There are significant medical-legal issues relating to interpretation of images that have been compressed for storage using a lossy algorithm where data are lost in the process.

- Because of the size of digital video files they must be compressed and are often transmitted in "streams," rather than as a single file.
- There are a number of compression/ decompression schemes that are used to convert digital video from a file to displayable format.
- Windows Media, Quicktime, and Real are three of the proprietary streaming formats that are common on the web.

Video images are increasingly used in patient care. Common examples include the recording of angiographic procedures such as coronary angiography or echocardiography. As with plain films, images from these procedures are now captured immediately to a digital format. Like digital plain films, digital video is of higher quality than its analog counterpart, does not degrade over time, is less expensive, faster to acquire and process, and is readily susceptible to enhancement techniques. Additionally, it is easy to arrange for remote viewing of a digital angiogram (over the internet) as contrasted to analog film.

The logistics relating to digital video management, as with much medical imaging, are formidable. Image sizes are typically 512×512 (or even 1024×1024) pixels, acquired at 30 frames/s (with at least 8 bits of resolution), and a typical procedure may be of the order of 5 min. Uncompressed the resulting file would be approximately 2.5 gigabytes of raw data. In order to transmit this over the Internet at a constant data rate of 64 Kbit/s it would take 80 hours. Even at 10 Mb/s it would take 30 min.

Table 16-3   Digital x-ray manipulation tools

Tool	Use
Pan	Move around image (with magnify)
Zoom	Enlarge or reduce image
Crop	Remove unnecessary parts of image
Magnify	Evaluate specific area (with pan)
Sharpness	Contrast enhancement
Smoothness	Eliminate noise
Window level	For specific tissues of interest
Measure	Precise measurements
Image inversion	To evaluate lines, tubes

It is clear that a system for transmitting angiogram video from one hospital to another requires a high bandwidth connection. Even then a wait of 30 min may be considered unacceptable, especially if a semi-real-time diagnosis is required. Compression may convert this from an impossible to a feasible process. Due to the sensitivity of the medical information however (as described above), only lossless or near-lossless algorithms can realistically be used. It is acceptable, for example, to have some degree of artifact in the video reproduction of an original newscast. The same degree of artifact may obscure or alter the diagnostic information in a digitally stored or transmitted angiogram.

There are a wide variety of video compression approaches in general use. The common theme, as with compression of still images, is the elimination of redundant information. In digital videos, there is typically only minimal change from one frame to the next, and the background in a given scene may remain totally unchanged for long periods if it is filmed from a fixed camera position. Video compression often involves two general steps. The first is intraframe compression, wherein a given frame of a digital video is compressed, and is similar conceptually to compression of still images. This is followed by interframe compression, which is applied to a sequence of video frames, rather than a single image (Fig. 16-10).

As with still compression, there are a variety of approaches to interframe compression. Subsampling simply removes frames from a sequence: every second or third frame might be removed with the assumption that the viewer's brain or an intelligent decoder (decompressor) will interpolate between the frames. Difference encoding is a process by which each frame of a sequence is compared with its predecessor and the only pixels that are updated are the ones that have change from their predecessor. Whereas difference encoding works on a pixel by pixel basis, block-based difference coding compares blocks of pixels from one frame to the next, and turns out to be a more efficient approach to compression than the pixel-based approach. There are other more sophisticated and efficient approaches to video compression that are beyond the scope of this book.

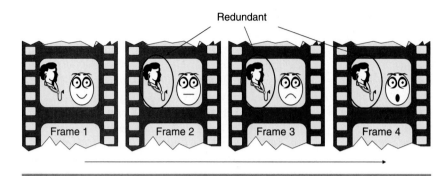

Figure 16-10
In video compression: (1) each frame is compressed and (2) information that remains unchanged from frame to frame is identified and handled efficiently so that there is both within and between frame compression.

One way of distributing medically oriented video content is to "burn" the content onto distribution media such as compact discs or DVDs. For example, it is very common to store studies such as coronary angiograms on CDs. If *web*-based delivery is to be used, the sender and the recipient must use the same "codec," which stands for compression/decompression scheme. There are two common approaches to the delivery of web video: streaming and downloading. When a file is downloaded, the process is fairly simple: the intended recipient typically "points at" the desired file on some web site and then downloads it into a file location on the local PC. That file can subsequently be viewed using the appropriate codec player at the recipient's convenience.

Streaming video is slightly more complicated. Streamed video is delivered to the recipient in a constant flow to the user's media player where it goes into a buffer. The media player begins to display the video when the buffer has enough data to tolerate fluctuations in flow from the Internet while still delivering constant flow to the player. Video streaming usually involves a third party "streaming media server" which can provide advanced delivery features such as fast recovery from stream interruptions (Fig. 16-11).

There are several well-recognized video formats with corresponding codecs that are prevalent on the Internet. These include Quicktime, Windows Media, RealVideo, and Flash Video. Quicktime is the Apple player and the one typically favored by professionals in the entertainment industry. Windows Media is the Microsoft codec and is bundled with Windows operating systems. RealVideo uses the Real proprietary format and while Real was an early entrant in the multimedia industry, it has given ground to the increasingly full featured, free competitors from Apple and Microsoft. Finally, the Flash codec from Macromedia is embedded in web browsers and increasingly popular for web-based

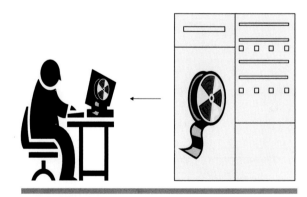

Figure 16-11
Medical video distribution.

video productions. Most of the aforementioned players will handle many video formats. The Windows Media Player, for example, will open and play most common video formats (although not the Real format).

Each of the players has specific nuances. The Quicktime player is obviously more prevalent on Apple machines, and is the preferred format in many user communities, such as the entertainment industry. The Windows Media Viewer is like many Microsoft products in that the early versions were unimpressive, but with time it has become the dominant player on the market as Microsoft has bundled it with its operating system software. The streaming video server (which provides video content to the Windows Media Viewer) is bundled with Windows Server (an operating system designed to run servers rather than user PCs). Real Video is both proprietary and more commercially oriented than the three other major competitors. The "free" Real viewer shows video with lower resolution than the purchased (Plus) version. Product installation is intrusive, associated with many unwanted product downloads, and the user is constantly "reminded" to upgrade the existing version of the product. The Flash player is increasingly the codec of choice for web programmers. Flash videos are viewed using software that is embedded in the browser and therefore don't open an additional window.

Conclusion

The electronic medical record of the future will not look like today's record nor will it be stored or transmitted in the same way. Digital creation, recording, and storage will radically change the way that information is packaged. It is very possible, for example, that "the medical record" will comprise component parts stored in a variety of locations. The radiographic data will likely be stored in one location, lab data in another, critical documents in a third. The record could be partially or fully assembled when needed. Still and moving images are already moving across the Internet for telemedicine applications and the extrapolation to "on demand" assembly of a medical record is intuitive.

Clinicians are increasingly required to work with and understand the implications of digitally stored medical information. The future, when telepresence and examination is common, will require a clear understanding of the benefits and consequences of digital medical data.

Suggested Readings

Symes P. *Digital Video Compression*. TAB/McGraw-Hill, 2003

Vaughan T. *Multimedia: Making it Work*, 6th ed. McGraw-Hill: Osbourne, 2003.

Compression Primer from Adobe: http://www.adobe.com/products/dvcoll/pdfs/DV_Compression_Primer.pdf.

Handheld Computing

Introduction

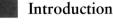

Key Points

- Clinicians are busier than ever before and time dedicated to information retrieval and documentations competes with the demands for direct patient care.
- Personal digital assistants (PDAs) and other portable computing devices with wireless capabilities are increasingly useful in medical care.
- PDAs can be used both as standalone devices or extensions of hospital networks.
- PDAs can facilitate the use of standardized best practices.
- Early data suggest that PDAs allow practitioners to be more efficient.

Clinicians are working harder: seeing more patients with less time and lower reimbursement. Tools that increase efficiency without affecting patient care are one answer to the need for greater efficiency, much as automated assembly lines helped to increase the efficiency of American industry in the 1980s and 1990s. Handheld computers of various sorts are increasingly popular both as standalone assistants and as wireless terminals carried by clinicians as part of a hospital information system. The latter obviously have substantially greater functionality to the degree that they allow information to flow from the clinician to the network and vice versa (Fig. 17-1).

Palm and Windows have differing operating systems for palm-sized devices (Fig. 17-2) and a number of software vendors have manufactured medical software designed to facilitate the jobs of clinicians as they practice. While the prototypical devices had black and white screens, newer models feature color screens, wireless capabilities, photography, and voice recording and playing. Small devices like these can be carried in a pocket, while larger computers such as a tablet PC are more analogous to a clipboard, albeit one with substantially enhanced abilities.

According to a recent study by Forrester's Consumer Technographics, clinicians are generally more technologically oriented than other consumers: online more often, more likely to own PDAs, have personal computers at home, have broadband connections at home and work, and use computers in the process of doing their job.

Many medical schools now mandate and subsidize the purchase of handheld devices, which have replaced the pocketful of quick reference guides carried by medical students and house officers in previous eras (Fig. 17-3). Programs such as patient trackers, drug databases, and medical references are ubiquitous both as free downloads and commercial products.

The PDA is well suited to medical applications because it is an electronic tool that acts at the point of care. There are several key drivers favoring the use of PDAs in clinical practice, including the rising costs of healthcare, increased demand for clinicians, increased demands on clinicians, advances in technology, and a growing awareness of medical errors. Significant gains in the efficiency of care can be realized by automating information acquisition by the clinician (i.e., handwriting normalization, preformatted text, prompts, protocol automation) and "pushing" information to the clinician (i.e., lab and radiology studies, email). The PDA can act also as a multipurpose pocket consultant. Finally, and perhaps most importantly, many believe that substantial

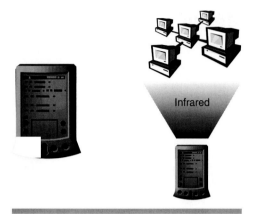

Figure 17-1
PDAs can function in either a standalone or networked configuration in a medical setting.

reductions in medical errors can be achieved by the use of PDAs at the point of care (Fig. 17-4).

Some recent survey data from a study of 900 clinicians, while admittedly unscientific, indicated that 20% used PDAs integrated with a network while 80% were used as standalones. Most of the respondents felt that the use of PDAs helped to improve the provision of care and reduce errors. Many felt that they were able to see two to three more patients per day than they would otherwise. Respondents used their PDAs for drug references, clinical references, and hospital guidelines most typically.

PDA Devices and Operating Systems

Key Points

- Apple pioneered the concept of the PDA with the Newton which sold poorly and wasn't quite portable enough.
- The Palm pilot was the first commercially successful PDA.
- Palm, Windows, and Research in Motion (which makes the Blackberry) are the major vendors of PDA operating systems today.
- There are a large number of devices and PDA capabilities are increasingly integrated with other functions, such as cell phones and cameras.

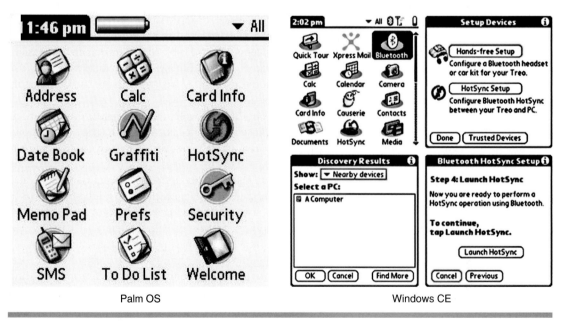

Figure 17-2
PDA operating systems.

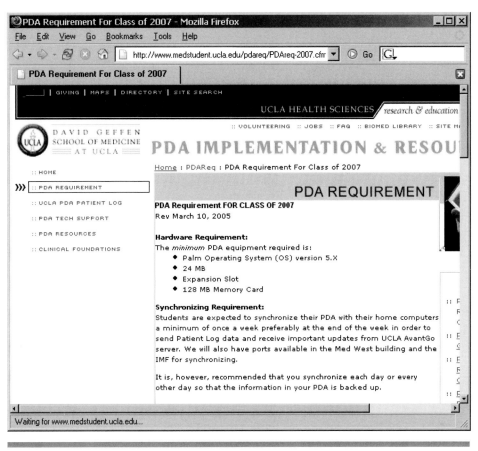

Figure 17-3
Many medical schools require the use of PDAs as part of the curriculum.

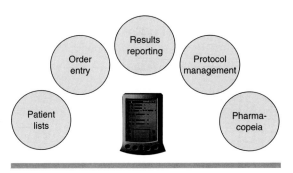

Figure 17-4
There are many potential uses of PDAs in the delivery of medical care.

During the sometimes-painful birth of the devices now called PDAs, several lessons became clear. The first is that size matters. Battery life matters as well. PDAs are not replacements for desktop computers, nor are their operating systems shrunken down versions of existing operating systems. Finally, they are not self-sufficient. PDAs function best when they act as extensions of the software commonly available on PCs, such as calendars, word processors, and so on.

The progenitor PDA was the Newton, which was presented to the marketplace in 1992 by the then CEO of Apple Computers John Scully. Apple's device was intended to capture, organize, and communicate information, and while it certainly captured the imagination of the public, it didn't sell. It featured handwriting recognition, albeit primitive, and other organization software such as notes, names, and dates. Its failure was attributed to its cost (over $1000) and the fact that it wasn't really a pocket portable device (Fig. 17-5).

The first successful PDA was the Palm pilot, which was released in 1996. It was a true PDA in that it was pocket ready, inexpensive, and multifunctional. It was also designed to synchronize with a PC, rather than acting purely as a standalone system, thereby permitting backups and software upgrades. The Palm operating system is designed to be fast and efficient so that software applications load and execute quickly and that underlying hardware is not overtaxed. Hardware choices also have implications for battery life, and the Palm devices have battery lives lasting weeks.

Windows entered the PDA market after Palm with the development of the Windows CE operating system. The initial Windows CE devices were far more powerful than Palm devices and had color screens. They integrated well with Windows operating systems and other Microsoft software such as

Table 17-1 Operating system comparison

	Palm	Windows CE
Size (smaller)	√	
Battery life	√	
Screen resolution/quality		√
Number of available medical applications	√	
Integrate with Windows applications		√
Expense (cheaper)	√	
Multitasking		√
Speed	√	

the Office suite. They were also typically more expensive and slower (Table 17-1).

Research in Motion's Blackberry devices are another form of PDA, although they typically are used purely for integration with an organization's office-oriented software, and medical applications are lacking. These devices can synchronize seamlessly with an enterprise mail server and calendaring system.

Today's market share for PDAs is divided up among Palm-based devices at about 40%, Windows CE devices at 40%, and Research in Motion devices. The most common products based on the Palm operating system are the Palm, Tungsten, Zire, CLIE, and Treo handhelds. The HP iPAQ pocket PC is probably the best-known Windows CE devices, although Dell sells a device called the Axim using a Windows OS as well. The devices sold by Research in Motion are the Blackberry family. Not all of these products are useful for the medical practitioner, who needs special software (Fig. 17-6).

PDAs in Medical Practice

Key Points

■ The traditional pocket medical information manager was the index card.

■ Information management is estimated to consume between 25 and 40% of a clinician's time.

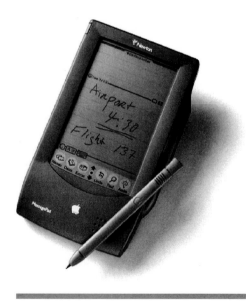

Figure 17-5
The Apple Newton.

- A variety of patient-specific tasks are susceptible to automation at the point of care including patient data forms, patient surveys, electronic disease diaries.

- Many clinician tasks are also well suited to automation with a PDA including patient lists, charge capture, results reporting, and decision support.

The traditional information management paradigm for the hospital-based practitioner is the maintenance of individual patient information on a series of 3 × 5 in. index cards clipped together in some fashion, with critical intake information as well as a series of cryptic notes relating to tasks. Paper lists of this sort are portable, easy to access, susceptible to quick data entry in any location, cheap and require no training to use. The disadvantages relate to issues such as limited space, inconsistent data entry among users (i.e., different annotations and handwriting).

It has been estimated that between 25 and 40% of a clinician's time is spent in administrative tasks such as data gathering and transcription. Many of these tasks can be automated cheaply, making clinicians much more efficient (Fig. 17-7). Some of the functions that have been automated include patient forms entry such as patient surveys, previsit screening

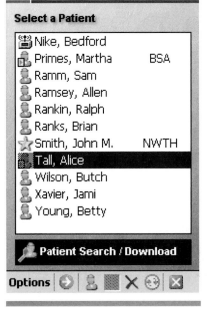

Figure 17-7
PDAs can be used to maintain patient lists.

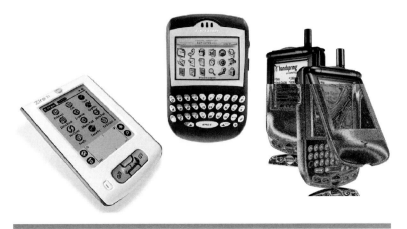

Figure 17-6
Various PDAs.

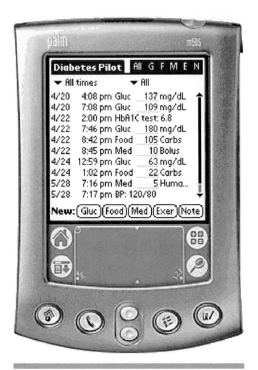

Figure 17-8
PDA-based patient logs can be used for
diabetes or asthma or for intake forms.

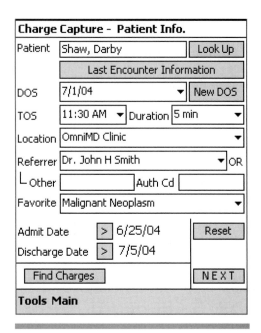

Figure 17-9
PDAs can be used for clinician charge
capture.

information acquisition, and electronic disease diaries (e.g., for asthma, diabetes) (Fig. 17-8).

There are several categories of clinician applications that are available from handheld software vendors. These include applications designed to address
administrative needs, the provision of clinical information, reference providers, and clinical tools.

The administrative applications include charge
capture, email communications, procedure logs.
Clinical information applications are represented by
results, order entry, medication lists, problem lists,
and consultations. There are also software applications providing drug and formulary tools, literature searches, and medical calculators (Figs. 17-9
to 17-11).

Charge capture applications are available from
several vendors to automate coding and patient
tracking for individual and groups of clinicians.
They use databases of ICD9 and CPT codes. Using

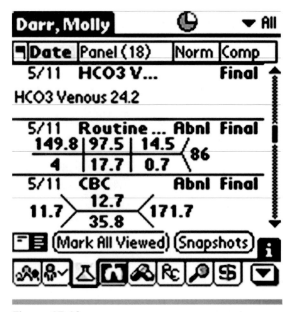

Figure 17-10
Patient results reporting.

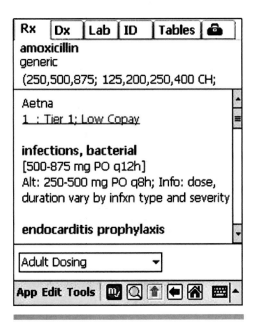

AIR	Transcutaneous Pacing
ANE	Transthoracic Pacing
CAR	Transvenous Pacing
ENT	Defibrillation
GAS	Elective Cardioversion
NEU	Emergency Cardioversion
OBG	Massage-Closed
ORT	Massage-Open
PLA	Cardiac Wound Repair
RAD	Pericardiocentesis
RES	Thoracentesis
URO	Thoracostomy-Needle
VAS	Thoracostomy-Tube

Figure 17-11
PDAs can act as portable formulary and
drug references.

Figure 17-12
Patient procedure logs can be used for
billing and competency documentation.

interfaces to the HIS patient location function, these
systems make it possible to quickly look up a patient
using any of variety of "tags," generate a charge,
and wirelessly upload it to servers. Email communications are an efficient way to communicate among
providers and are part of the functionality of several
of the available PDAs. Many residents, medical
interventionalists, and surgeons maintain procedure
logs for administrative purposes using software
designed for this purpose (Fig. 17-12).

Tools designed to enhance the delivery of care
can significantly increase the efficiency of a mobile
provider. Automated communication of results with
or without alerts and order entry using a wireless
link to the HIS eliminates the needed to find a hospital terminal. These activities can occur in the background as the clinician moves about the hospital. A
PDA can also be used to maintain patient problem
lists, tasks, notes, medication lists, and histories.

Finally, PDAs are often used as portable references, (Fig. 17-13) allowing a clinician to carry the

equivalent of several critical reference texts in a
pocket. Drug references and clinical texts are available from several vendors. The information in
these texts can be kept up-to-date by synchronizing
the PDA with central servers on a regular basis.
Some hospitals have used PDAs as a mechanism to
enhance the use of formulary drugs, and to minimize drug costs by intervening at the point of drug
prescribing with decision support messages suggesting the least costly, appropriate choice of
therapies. Other hospital-specific information,
such as guidelines and protocols endorsed by that
institution can be outlined on a PDA, which has
the combined effect of enhancing compliance and
supporting the clinician in the provision of care.

Alternative Technologies

Key Points

- There are other handheld or portable devices that
  a clinician can use at the point of care, such as
  tablet PCs.

- Wearable computers are likely to become
  available in the near future with novel interface
  devices, like eyeglass-based displays and voice
  interfaces.

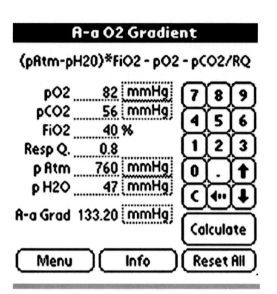

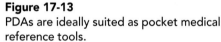

Figure 17-13
PDAs are ideally suited as pocket medical reference tools.

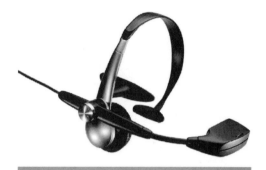

Figure 17-14
The next generation of portable medical tools will use new tools to permit continuous hands-free interaction with wearable computers.

Handheld solutions and functionality will undoubtedly continue to improve, just as PC technology has. There are other alternatives currently available and on the near horizon as well. The tablet PC represents an attractive alternative to a laptop in that it can use a number of data entry approaches, including handwriting, has the full functionality of a laptop, and is light enough to carry.

A technology that is not yet commercially available but will be within the very near future is wearable computers. What the form factor will ultimately look like is unclear. Some demonstration projects have integrated the circuitry into plates worn on the torso, others into a fanny pack. The monitor can be built into eyeglasses and use a head's up (see through) or head-mounted (projection) display (Fig. 17-14). Alternatively, body-mounted displays and handheld displays area available using smaller, liquid crystal displays. Interface technologies include voice, special keyboards, wrist-mounted keyboards, and mice.

Wearable technologies could replace handheld devices during the provision of routine medical care. It is easy to imagine unique uses as well. For example, image guided surgery currently uses data sets loaded into a display system that superimposes the image of the instrument on the radiographic image. Similarly, laparoscopic surgery uses displays positioned at the side of the surgical table. A wearable computer and display could significantly assist the operator. Additionally, the operator could "call up" images or data to the computer he's wearing during the course of a procedure. A cardiac surgeon engaged in a coronary artery bypass operation might wish, for example, to review the patient's coronary an-atomy during the course of a procedure. Using a head-mounted device wirelessly attached to the hospital's radiology system, he could do so without ever scrubbing out. A telemedicine consultant could handle urgent consultations from any location with wireless access to the Internet, which will soon include many urban environments. This presupposes, of course, that the right security and privacy mechanisms are in place.

Conclusion

A useful analogy to the changes in medicine that will ultimately result from widespread deployment of portable computing is the enormous societal changes that have resulted from cellular telephony. For better or worse, the portability and immediacy of cellular phone access have changed the way people interact, as is immediately apparent wherever people gather. The addition of still and video camera technology to cell phones will, no doubt, have additional consequences. Medical practice will undergo similar, albeit still unclear, changes as the computing interface evolves from a fixed location to an "always-on," mobile paradigm.

Suggested Readings

Papadakis MA, McPhee SJ, Tierney LM. *CURRENT DxTx Ready Reference for PDA : Clinical Highlights from CURRENT Medical Diagnosis & Treatment.* New York: McGraw-Hill, 2003.

American Medical Student Association: http://www.amsa.org/resource/pda.cfm.

PDAMD.com: http://www.pdamd.com/vertical/tutorials/buyersguide.xml.

CHAPTER 18

Implanted Biochips

Introduction

Key Points

■ Implanted computer chips have been the subject of science fiction for many years.

■ New developments in imaging, hardware, and our understanding of the physiology and pathophysiology of the brain and the organs it innervates have resulted in significant developments in the use of implanted computers.

"The matrix has its roots in primitive arcade games in early graphics programs and military experimentation with cranial jacks." *Neuromancer*

Neuromancer was published in 1984 (Fig. 18-1). Its author, William Gibson, is regarded as a cyberpunk visionary who described a networked world in which people "jack in" to Gibson's Internet, which he called the Matrix, using a direct connection to the brain. The "cranial jack," "dermatrodes," "nervesplicing," and "micro bionics" are interface technologies described in the book permitting direct linkage between the brain and the electronic medium. This is rightly regarded as a seminal novel, but it is in an earlier novel by another visionary that we see one of the first references to bioelectronic interfaces.

Michael Crichton's *The Terminal Man* was published in 1972, and is about a man with recurrent seizures who enrolls in a scientific experiment in which terminals are implanted in his brain. The protagonist, Harry, is a computer programmer subject to murderous impulses which are brought on by "thought seizures." In order to rid himself of this troublesome problem, he has 40 electrodes implanted in the pleasure centers of his brain which, when activated, abort the seizures—at least

for a while, until things get really interesting (Fig. 18-2).

Interface, published in 1997 by Stephen Bury (the pen name for Neal Stephenson and J. Frederick George), marries the concepts of Gibson and Crichton with the strategies of the Clintons' White House. In it, a presidential candidate is implanted with a neural biochip through which he is directly interfaced to poll results. Needless to say, this gives him a leg up on the competition (Fig. 18-3).

While the ideas proposed by these authors were pure science fiction when they were written, reality is about to catch up. Neurosurgeons treat epilepsy by ablating seizure foci deep in the brain. Neural prostheses are being developed at a number of centers, and cochlear, retinal, and deep brain implants are under development. The National Institutes of Health (NIH) and the Defense Advanced Research Projects Agency (DARPA) are both funding work on neural devices including auditory and visual prostheses, diaphragmatic pacemakers (for patients like Christopher Reeves), and motor, bladder, or spinal cord stimulators.

Auditory Prostheses

Key Points

■ Hearing loss is usually categorized as being either conductive or sensorineural.

■ Conductive hearing loss results from damage to the "hardware" that conducts sound to the cochlea where it is translated into a neural signal.

■ Sensorineural hearing loss, which is most common, results from damage somewhere along the pathway from the cochlea to the auditory centers of the brain.

- Cochlear implants use an electrode to carry sound signals from an external microphone to the auditory nerve.
- Auditory implants bypass the auditory nerve and carry signals directly to the auditory centers in the brain.

Human hearing can be impaired at several levels, and it's useful to understand the functional anatomy of the ear. The ear itself is a cartilaginous structure designed to funnel sounds into the ear canal. Once a sound, which is actually vibration of the air molecules, reaches the eardrum, it too begins to vibrate. The eardrum is connected to the three bones of the

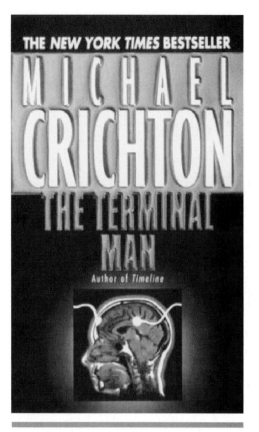

Figure 18-2
Michael Crichton's book describes a man with a neurally implanted pacemaker.

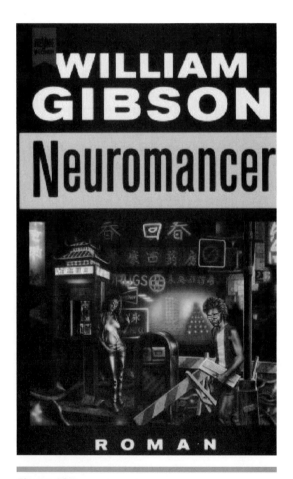

Figure 18-1
Gibson's Neuromancer is a classic sci-fi text in which he describes "the matrix."

middle ear, which are themselves connected to the cochlea, a fluid containing, seashell-like organ that is lined with sensitive hairs. The sound wave that hit the eardrum is converted to a fluid wave in the cochlea and the cochlear hairs sense the back and forth movement of the fluid. As the hairs move, they send signals to the hearing nerve about the frequency and amplitude of the wave. The hearing nerve (auditory nerve) carries this information to the brain, which integrates information about the sound from the two ears (thereby gaining directional information based on timing discrepancies).

Deafness can occur for a variety of reasons, but the most common is sensorineural deafness, in which some part of the inner ear (including the cochlea, hair cells, or auditory nerve) is damaged or

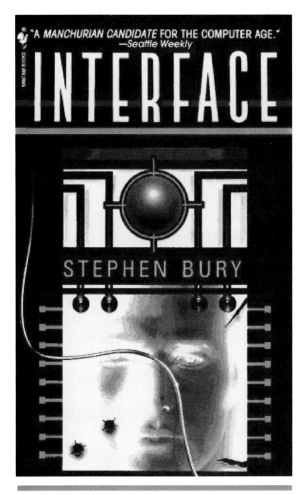

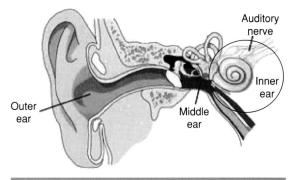

Figure 18-4
Sensorineural hearing loss involves damage to the cochlea or auditory nerve.

of cochlear hairs due to high decibel noise. Between 1971 and 1990, the number of people between the ages of 46 and 64 with hearing loss increased 26%, and the number between the ages of 18 and 44 increased 17%, according to the National Health Interview Survey (Fig. 18-5).

Whereas conductive hearing loss can often be treated surgically, sensorineural hearing loss typically requires the use of a prosthesis. Cochlear implants work by capturing sound with an external microphone, preprocessing it, and sending it by radio waves to an electrode implanted in the cochlea which, in turn, sends signals to the auditory nerve.

Figure 18-3
Interface describes a politician implanted with a wireless network interface giving him instantaneous polling information.

destroyed. This is often acquired, rather than hereditary, and can be due to aging, disease, infection, or damage from loud or constant noise (Fig. 18-4).

The other major form of deafness is conductive hearing loss resulting from injury or damage to the auditory canal (e.g., a foreign body such as wax or a pea), the eardrum (e.g., ruptured drum), the middle ear (e.g., fluid or pus in the middle ear), or the bones (ossicles) of the ear.

An increasingly common cause of acquired deafness in the "baby-boomer" generation is loss

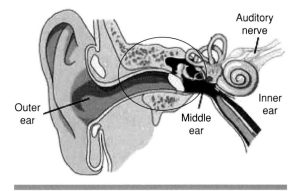

Figure 18-5
Conductive hearing loss involves damage to the eardrum or the bones that conduct sound to the cochlea.

As such, they bypass all of the components from the ear to the auditory nerve and could be used for most forms of deafness. Because they require a surgical procedure for implantation, and therefore carry the risks associated with the surgery and the implantation of a foreign body, they are not typically used for deafness that is amenable to treatment with a standard hearing aid (Fig. 18-6).

The most severe form of sensorineural deafness, in which the auditory nerve is destroyed or surgically removed, was previously untreatable because there was no way to carry information about sound to the brain. This problem has been partially solved by the development of the auditory brain implant, in which an electrode is placed in the brain, next to the portion of the brain responsible for hearing (the cochlear nucleus).

The cochlear implant and auditory brain implants of today are remarkable advances over the devices of 5 and 10 years ago. They are smaller and provide the patient with near normal speech recognition. The technology is advancing so rapidly, however, that descriptions of the latest technologies are almost immediately obsolete.

It is important to note, however, that both the cochlear implant and the auditory brain implant consist of both an implanted electrode or array of electrodes and an external device in which the sound

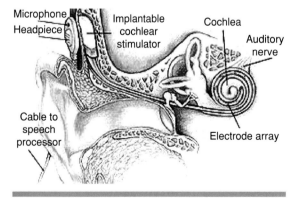

Figure 18-6
A cochlear implant combines an implanted stimulator with an external microphone and speech processing hardware.

is preprocessed for optimal recognition. The latter is obviously susceptible to easy modernization as hardware is miniaturized and improved. One can imagine an external appliance (consisting of the microphone and preprocessor) that can translate from one language to another on the fly, thereby providing the auditory bioprosthesis with capabilities unavailable to the unilingual individual with normal hearing. Similarly, an auditory bioprosthesis might be capable of picking up sounds that would be inaudible to humans with normal hearing—a dog's whistle, for example.

Visual Prostheses

Key Points

- The "eye" has developed independently at many points on the phylogenic tree.
- External visual prostheses have been around for a while.
- Bioelectronic visual prostheses are far behind their auditory counterparts, but an active area of research.

The eye is one of Mother Nature's most remarkable creations and one of which she was obviously quite proud. Much as Degas did with the female nude, Mother Nature kept tinkering with the eye as we can see from her experiments with mammals, insects, and shellfish, all of which have some, albeit very different, form of functional vision. The first human visual prosthesis were some form of spectacles, the origins of which are debated (some say the Far East some say the West) but certainly date back to the thirteenth or fourteenth century. Benjamin Franklin created the first bifocals, and Adolf Fick, a German physiologist, invented the first contact lens in the latter part of the nineteenth century. While much has been done with applied prostheses, and one can actually turn one's "brown eyes blue" with colored contact lenses, bioelectronic vision is in its infancy.

As with auditory prostheses, visual bioelectronic devices can be inserted at the end organ—the eye in this instance—or at the mother of all motherboards, the brain. The configuration of both, at least as currently conceived, is analogous to the auditory bioprostheses. There is an external *receptor* (a camera mounted on a pair of glasses) that acquires the sensory information and preprocesses it. The information is then relayed to an implanted device somewhere along the visual pathway.

The locations currently under evaluation for electronic *delivery* of visual information include intraocular sites in front of or behind the retina, points along the optic nerve, and directly into the visual areas of the brain (including the lateral geniculate body and the visual cortex). The implanted bioelectrode generates impulses that are relayed to or directly processed by the brain. The whole package comes alarmingly close to the artificial vision of Geordi La Forge, the blind pilot in Star Trek: The Next Generation (Fig. 18-7).

An obvious question pertains to the coding of the visual information acquired by the camera, and its perceived shape and orientation in the brain. The picture presented to a newly blind individual would presumably be formatted differently from the way in which the same view would have

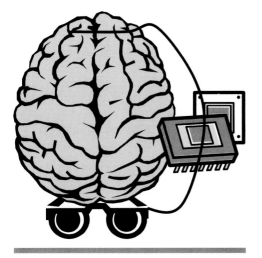

Figure 18-7
A visual bioprosthesis may involve acquisition of visual information using glasses which are connected to a visual processing unit and then to the brain.

been experienced with prior to the development of blindness. One could imagine the artificial scene being sideways or upside down relative to the real one, and certainly much sparser in detail. It turns out, however, that the adult visual cortex is amazingly adaptive.

When equipped with prism glasses that reversed their vision, a group of students in a Japanese study adapted to point that they were able to ride a bicycle (with the reversed visual field) after a month. Brain scans suggested that the brain accommodated by accepting the new perspective as a new reality rather than by attempting to translate to the old perspective on the fly. Test subjects are able to navigate and read with a very minimal visual input array of 25 × 25 pixels—which corresponds to the resolution of some of the very earliest computer monitors.

Visual bioprostheses are 5–10 years off by most estimates and are not expected, at first, to restore anything like normal vision. There is no reason, however, that the camera used in functional visual prosthesis couldn't be equipped to "see" wavelengths of light that a sighted human can't, such as infrared or ultraviolet, and therefore provide an analogue of "x-ray vision," admittedly at low resolution. Many of us remember the old ads for glasses in magazines aimed at male teenagers for glasses that would allow you to "See Through Women's Clothing." In fact, new airport scanners are becoming available that can do just that using *backscatter imaging*. While visual bioprostheses probably won't equip one to see through women's or men's clothing, they might allow a blind person to see warm objects at night that would be invisible to a sighted person or to see the ultraviolet wavelengths that are visible to birds and bees, but not us.

Pacemakers and Implantable Defibrillators

Key Points

- Cardiac pacemakers have been around for decades.
- Newer pacemakers are very intelligent, programmable, and can be triggered to pace or intervene in a number of ways.

- Cardiac pacemakers/defibrillators are able to identify and treat cardiac dysrythmias in a variety of ways.
- Phrenic pacemakers may soon free certain ventilator-dependent patients from the need for mechanical ventilation.

Cardiac Pacemakers

Cardiac pacemakers are probably the most widely deployed bioprostheses, and their evolution from primitive, single heart rate, clunky boxes to sophisticated, computers that can vary heart rate depending on need and sense and treat dysrhythmias is what we can assume will occur with auditory and visual devices.

Today's pacemakers are smaller than their predecessors, more efficient in terms of energy consumption, and smarter (Fig. 18-8). Small programmable pacemaker computers combined with bipolar (or multipolar) lead systems allow the use of hysteresis (which relates intrinsic heart rate to programmed heart rate), multiple-chamber pacing, multiple programmability, rate-adaptive pacing capabilities, and antitachycardia pacing. Rate-adaptive pacemakers can sense body movement, for example, and increase heart rate, based on the assumption that increased movement implies exercise and increased demand. An obvious problem with that assumption occurs when the body is subjected to external sources of movement such as those experienced during a bumpy car ride. An alternative approach to increasing heart rate based on "demand" is to modulate the paced rate based on respiratory rate.

The implantable pacemaker/cardio-defibrillator (ICD) is larger and more electrically powerful than a pacemaker (Fig. 18-9). It is a sophisticated, complex rhythm management device. Its defibrillating circuitry can be programmed to deliver low energy (1–5 J) to terminate ventricular tachycardia at moderate rates or higher energy (10–40 J) to terminate rapid, polymorphic tachycardia and ventricular fibrillation. Moderate rate ventricular tachycardia can be terminated by burst pacing through the ventricular pacing circuit rather than (or before attempting) defibrillation.

The ICDs pacemaker circuitry is capable of the same programmable pacing options as offered by

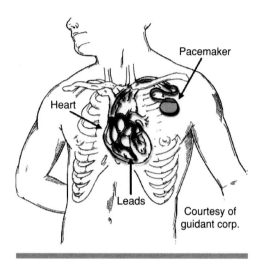

Figure 18-8
Pacemakers are small computers that use information from the heart and respond accordingly.

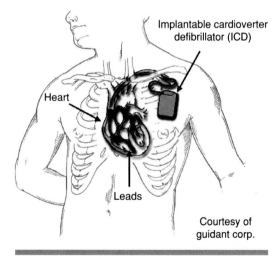

Figure 18-9
An automatic implantable defibrillator can function as a pacemaker as well as deliver a defibrillatory shock to the heart when needed.

modern pacemakers. Single, dual, biventricular, and sensor-mediated pacing are possible, and in fact essential after defibrillation. Some ICDs can be programmed to terminate atrial fibrillation or flutter using rapid atrial pacing or by delivering defibrillation energy.

Recent data have shown that biventricular pacing is effective as a treatment in heart failure. Because of all of the foregoing applications and data, the use of implantable pacemakers and defibrillators is increasing.

Smart pacemakers can also communicate with hospital-based units over the phones, giving doctors a quick way of interrogating the pacemaker and diagnosing problems.

Pacemaker manufacturers are developing smarter algorithms, and expect that pacemakers will eventually be sewn directly onto or into the heart and become susceptible to the body's intrinsic messages regulating heart rate, such as the fight or flight reaction.

Phrenic Pacemakers

The diaphragm is controlled by a nerve called the *phrenic* nerve which, like all other peripheral nerves, derives from the spinal cord. The word derives from the Greek root meaning diaphragm and also mind, and relates to the fact that the Greeks believed that the characteristically human part of the mind resides in the diaphragm. Interestingly, breathing is usually automatic and subconscious, yet it can also be controlled willfully, or its perception can rise, uncomfortably in many cases, to the level of consciousness.

Injuries to the phrenic nerve, or to the high spinal cord in the neck, interrupt breathing resulting in death within minutes. Christopher Reeves, the actor, and Stephen Hawking, the theoretical physicist, both suffer from different forms of injuries to the nerves that control breathing, traumatic in Reeve's case and Lou Gehrig's disease in the second. Both of these men have been totally dependent on ventilators, with their inherent risks and limitations. Reeves was actually able to be freed from the ventilator for periods after implantation of a phrenic pacemaker prior to his death in the Fall of 2004 (Fig. 18-10).

Unfortunately, and for a variety of reasons, diaphragmatic pacers are employed infrequently. This relates in part to the fact that a more invasive surgical procedure is required to implant a diaphragmatic pacer that a cardiac pacer, and probably to the fact that the market for diaphragmatic pacers is considerably smaller than that for cardiac pacemakers. Patients who have undergone diaphragmatic pacemaker placement are able to speak, are more mobile than those on ventilators, may have lower infection rates and improved satisfaction.

Bladder Pacemakers

Another set of muscles susceptible to pacing are those that control the bladder. Patients with spinal cord injuries, and other diseases (such as multiple sclerosis) are unable to sense fullness in the bladder

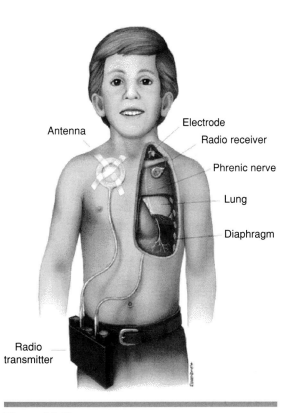

Antenna

Electrode
Radio receiver
Phrenic nerve
Lung
Diaphragm

Radio transmitter

Figure 18-10
Phrenic pacemakers are used for patients with cervical injuries.

and frequently develop bladder infections due to the need for intermittent catheterization of the bladder. Other patients suffer from incontinence, urgency, or frequency. Using a technology similar to that of the diaphragmatic pacer, with an implanted receiver and a transcutaneous transmitter, the bladder can be stimulated to empty on demand. Like the diaphragmatic pacer, however, bladder pacing necessitates a rather involved surgical procedure to place the stimulating electrodes.

Many of the difficulties associated with placement of electrodes are likely to be alleviated by the development and widespread application of laparoscopic techniques. Diaphragmatic muscle stimulation can be performed with stimulating electrodes placed laparoscopically. With the ongoing evolution of surgery through a scope, small incisions and miniaturization of electronic components, diaphragmatic and bladder pacing are likely to come into greater use, freeing spinal cord injured patients from some of the constraints and risks associated with current management approaches.

Deep Brain Stimulation

Implanted electrodes are also being used to alleviate symptoms of depression, obsessive-compulsive disease, Parkinson's disease, and other nervous system movement disorders. A new FDA-approved electrical stimulation device involves a combination of wires implanted in the brain using stereotaxic surgery and an attached, programmable pulse generator. The deep brain stimulation (DBS) device, very similar to a cardiac pacemaker, is being implanted at several centers with promising results (Fig. 18-11).

The pulse generator is initially programmed with feedback from positron emission tomography (PET), and subsequently adjusted based on clinical results, objective tests, and further PET scanning.

Robotic Implants

There are a number of microchip technologies specifically designed for patients with injuries to the spinal cord, peripheral nervous system, and extremities.

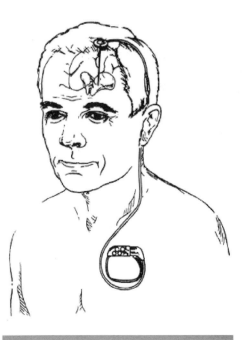

Figure 18-11
Deep brain pacemaker stimulation is being used for treatment of depression and Parkinson's disease.

The term functional electrical stimulation (FES) is used to describe approaches to restoring limb function after nerve injury using electrodes. Some of the projects that come under the aegis of FES include systems in which an implanted sensor in the wrist or shoulder is used to generate signals controlling the contraction of the muscles in the hand. More radical approaches are being investigated wherein the mere thought or visualization of a hand movement might be translated into the appropriate movement.

Conclusion

Implanted computers are increasingly prevalent and effective for the treatment of a variety of disease states. Circuitry is shrinking in size at the same rate as circuitry in other computing devices (as predicted by Moore's Law), and devices may soon be small enough to eliminate the need for wired attachments. Increasingly sophisticated algorithms can be used for treatment, and external reprogramming is routine. The science fiction fantasies of Gibson, Crichton, and Stephenson have become reality and we may soon see the day when we can "jack" directly into the Matrix.

Suggested Readings

Perkowitz S. *Digital People: From Bionic Humans to Androids*. Joseph Henry Press, Washington DC; 2004.

Geary J. *The Body Electric: An Anatomy of the New Bionic Senses*. Rutgers University Press, New Jersey; 2002.

CHAPTER 19

Artificial Intelligence and Robotics

 Introduction

Key Points

- Medicine is a labor-intensive industry that lags behind other nonfarm industries in productivity.
- Automation using intelligent software and robotics is an obvious solution but one which faces regulatory and labor force resistance.
- The automation of the airline cockpit has many instructive parallels for the medical industry.

Medicine is a labor-intensive industry with a relatively low investment in computers and technology. When compared to other industries, the rate of labor productivity growth in the hospital sector lags well behind the nonfarm sector. As medical costs continue to escalate, pressures for cost-efficiencies and increased productivity will continue to grow (Fig. 19-1).

There are a number of ways in which medical care is bound to practice models (i.e., specific nursing ratios for ICU patients) that could be streamlined, but will be difficult to change. For example, it is easy to imagine ways in which care in an ICU or operating room could be made more efficient and less labor-intensive using intelligent computer algorithms and/or robotics. In much the same way that airline cockpits have become automated using intelligent software and fly-by-wire technology, some of the activities of ICU and operating room nurses and physicians could be performed by machines. Automation of the cockpit permitted a reduction in crew size.

The crew manning commercial long-haul aircraft in the 1950s consisted of five to six people, including two pilots (plus a relief pilot), a flight engineer, navigator, and radio operator. The latter role was folded into that of the pilots fairly quickly, and the role of the navigator was eliminated in the 1970s with the advent of new navigation technology. The flight engineer remained part of the crew until the mid-1980s, when the 747 became available, with computers that performed many of the tasks previously done by the engineer. The battle over the elimination of the "third man" (the engineer) is instructive. Pilots unions fought automation fiercely, and it wasn't until a presidential commission endorsed the conversion to two man cockpits that the change became possible (Table 19-1).

The evolution of the automated cockpit is instructive. The engineers who designed the automated cockpit were initially concerned that pilots would have too little work in the new cockpits. It quickly became apparent, however, that automation created new work relating to interaction between the pilots and the computers. Too much information was presented to the pilots in early cockpit software, distracting them from important functions such as scanning the local sky for other planes. Human factors research evolved to address issues relating to the interaction between people and machines.

Returning to the medical environment, many of the tasks performed by medical clinicians could be automated or made easier through the use of new technologies that have been well tested in other industries. Robotics has enhanced the productivity and quality of products once made on human

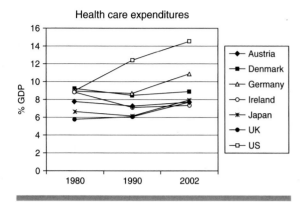

Figure 19-1
Medical costs as a percentage of gross domestic product are escalating at an unsustainable pace.

Table 19-1 Cockpit personnel for transoceanic flight

Year	Crew Size	Crew Members
1950s	5–6	2 pilots, (relief pilot), engineer, navigator, radio operator
1960s	4–5	2 pilots, (relief pilot), engineer, navigator
1970s	3–4	2 pilots, (relief pilot), engineer
1980s	2–3	2 pilots, (relief pilot)

assembly lines. Tasks once felt to be so critical that only a human pilot could perform them (takeoff, landing) are now routinely delegated to computer programs. Analogously, many of the documentation, titration, and analytic tasks performed by ICU nurses and anesthesia providers could be automated with resulting improvements in efficiency and quality.

◼ Intelligent Medical Software

Key Points

◼ Vast quantities of medical data are being acquired electronically and very little of it is examined for useful information.

◼ New software tools are available that can be used to "mine" medical data.

◼ Data mining can be defined as the process of (automatically) extracting previously unknown, valid and actionable information from large databases and using the information to make crucial medical decisions.

◼ Neural networks (NNs), genetic algorithms (GAs), belief networks, fuzzy logic, and data visualization are some of the tools that can be brought to bear on the analysis of medical data.

The amount of data acquired electronically from patients has grown exponentially during the past decade. Hospital databases including demographic systems, electronic patient records, as well as order-entry, laboratory, pharmacy, and radiology systems grow in scope and data capacity with each year. Modern bedside monitors communicate with a host of devices through data busses and interchangeable, plug-in interfaces. Bedside equipment stores electronic data, huge databases have been acquired by insurers and governments containing demographic-, procedural-, and disease-specific information.

In its raw form, data are relatively uninformative. Handled properly, however, data can be mined for novel and unexpected information (Fig. 19-2). Computer science has developed a number of new tools to extract information from data and enhance analysis by the human clinical expert. In many cases, these new tools are modeled on physiologic processes, such as human cognition (neural network, case-based reasoning) or human reproduction genetic algorithm.

Terminology

It is useful to begin by defining several terms used commonly in describing computer systems used for data analysis. The appropriate definition of *artificial intelligence* (AI) is controversial. Alan Turing, the English mathematician, devised what has become known as the Turing test of computer intelligence. He suggested that a computer had AI if it could successfully mimic a human and thereby fool another human. An *expert system* is a computer program that simulates the judgment and behavior of a human or an organization with expert knowledge and experience in a particular field. *Data mining* is

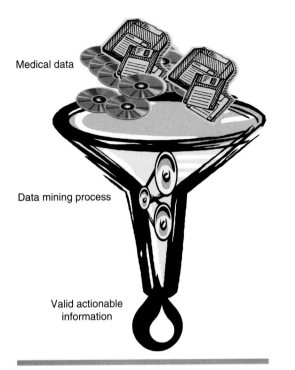

Medical data

Data mining process

Valid actionable
information

Figure 19-2
Data mining is the process of (automatically)
extracting previously unknown, valid and
actionable information from large databases, and
using the information to make crucial decisions.

the analysis of data for relationships that have not
previously been discovered. Techniques used for
data mining can discover hidden associations or
sequences in data sets, clustering of data points, and
permit visualization of relationships among data or
forecasting based on hidden patterns. Data mining is
also known as knowledge discovery, and derives its
roots from statistics, AI, and machine learning. A
data warehouse is a central repository for all or significant parts of the data that an enterprise's (read
hospital information system) systems collect. An
alternative term is a *data mart*.

The concept of medical expert systems has been
around since the advent of AI in the 1960s and
1970s. However, clinicians have been reluctant to
integrate computerized data analysis tools into
their practice in part due to the failed promise of
early expert systems.

Early AI systems were rule-based systems,
which can be thought of as "top-down" systems,
which begin with a complex model and use a
reductionist approach to simulate a process pro-
grammatically. Reductionism breaks a problem
down into its constituent parts to arrive at the
essential components that characterize it. This
approach can be used to model the way in which
an expert clinician thinks or acts. In reality, however, experts make rapid, often intuitive, decisions
beginning with a few hypotheses selected by experience, followed by clinical or laboratory observations that further refine the differential diagnosis.
When asked to explain their thinking, many experts
are unable to coherently explain the process by
which they arrived at a diagnosis.

Early Rule-Based Systems

Two of the first AI systems in medicine were the
MYCIN infectious disease consultant program
Internist system described in Chap. 11. Both of these
were rule-based systems and both demonstrated
academic success. Neither, however, has survived to
the present day. One pioneer in medical computing,
Enrico Coiera, has said: "Artificial intelligence in
medicine (AIM) has not been successful if success is
judged as making an impact on the practice of medicine. Much recent work in AIM has been focused
inward (sic), addressing problems that are at the
crossroads of the parent disciplines of medicine and
AI. Now, AIM must move forward with the insights
that it has gained and focus on finding solutions for
problems at the heart of medical practice."

There are many factors that have slowed the
acceptance of AI solutions in medicine, including the
small margin for error in medical decision making
and the ready availability of experts in many environments. These obstacles are likely to change in the
near term, as computer solutions improve, performance pressures increase, and the number of experts
dwindles. To the extent that computer-based tools
can act as clinician extenders, they will become
increasingly acceptable.

Unlike the previous generation of AI tools,
newer tools are data-driven, and take advantage
of the fact that large databases can be mined to

"discover" relationships among the data elements. They assume that patterns discerned from this kind of analysis can be used to predict the future behavior of the systems that generated the old data. Unlike the prior generation of top-down systems, newer systems are "bottom up," in which the data generated by the system can be used to characterize the system (Fig. 19-3). An analogous business example might be the derivation of the probability of mortgage default based on a large demographic data set of prior applicants. The bottom-up tools are cheaper to build and easier to maintain than their predecessors.

Model-Driven Versus Data-Driven AI

It is useful to contrast the model-driven and data-driven systems using a familiar physiologic example. A top-down, rule-based AI model would have rules about the relationship between pulmonary artery occlusion pressure (PAOP) and cardiac output (CO) based upon well-accepted physiologic principles such as the Frank-Starling mechanism, whereas a bottom-up system would have no "preconceptions." Instead, the latter would analyze a large body of observations about the relationship between PAOP and CO in a given patient and derive that patient's Frank-Starling relationship.

Note that the top-down approach embodies general rules about all patients: "If the PAOP is less than or equal to 5 mmHg and if the CO is less than 2 L/min then give fluid bolus" Conversely, the bottom-up approach is used to discover the physiologic behavior of one individual from data acquired during continuous monitoring of that patient: "When Mr. Jones' PAOP decreases to less than 8 mmHg, his CO decreases to less than 3 L/min." The former imposes structure on the data, whereas the latter derives structure from the data.

Data mining evolved from previous generations of data analysis tools, and several different techniques are in common use in data mining, or data-driven

Expert system rule

| If (patient has a low K⁺) and (patient is (not) on beta blocker) then (probability of atrial fibrillation is increased) |

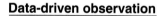

Data-driven observation

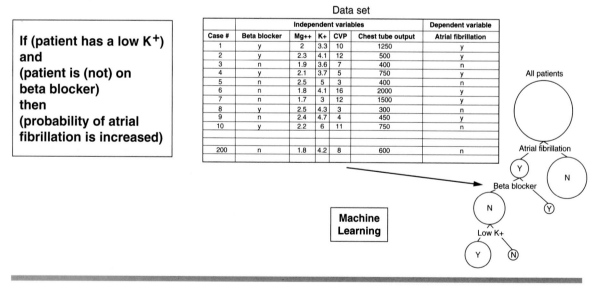

Figure 19-3
The expert system (top-down) vs. data-driven (bottom-up) approaches may arrive at the same conclusion, but the latter is self-teaching and requires little maintenance.

decision support. They include NNs, GAs, Bayesian or belief networks, rule induction or case-based reasoning, and machine learning. Fuzzy logic is a relatively new approach to programming that permits ambiguity in descriptions of data. Data visualization techniques are used to display large amounts of data in a way that permits recognition of relationships among the elements.

Neural Networks

Neural networks are intended to mimic the mechanisms of the human brain. NNs consist of input nodes (or neurodes), output nodes, and internal (or hidden) nodes or layers. The nodes are connected with different architectures, but typically input nodes are connected to hidden layer nodes and they are in turn connected to output nodes. The neural network analyzes (or trains on) a data set to find clusters of outputs or relationships among input and output elements. During this process, the relative importance of (or weights of) connections between nodes are adjusted. In effect, important connections are reinforced (positively weighted) and unimportant connections are punished (negatively weighted). Data are fed into the input nodes, processed through the hidden layer(s), and the connection weights to the output nodes are adjusted (Fig. 19-4).

Neural nets are categorized based on the way that they analyze data. In supervised networks, the outputs are known but the importance of the relationship of a given input to an output is unknown prior to training. In unsupervised networks, the outputs are unknown and the system is encouraged to find interesting, often unsuspected, relationships among the data elements in large data sets, which typically present as clusters of data. For example, in mining a state's Medicare database with an unsupervised neural network, one might discover an unexpected cluster of postoperative surgical deaths at a given hospital or a cluster of specific malignancies in a particular geographic region. The major weakness in neural network solutions is the fact that the methods by which a relationship is discovered are hidden (or

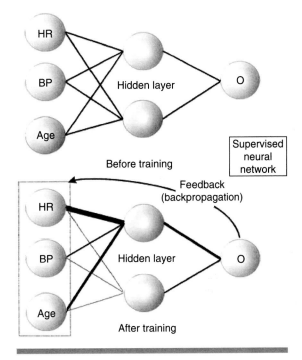

Figure 19-4
Supervised neural networks analyze the relationships among data elements and, with feedback, can be "trained" to recognize patterns of interest.

opaque) and therefore not readily understood or explained.

Genetic Algorithms

Genetic algorithms are modeled on the principles of Darwinian selection, and designed to find near optimal solutions to complicated problems. For example, GAs have been used to find a near optimal solution to the so-called traveling salesman problem, which was once considered unsolvable as the number of cities became very large. GAs can provide a best approximation. The process involves (1) the creation of a number of possible solutions, (2) competition among them using selection criteria (i.e., fastest route, least expensive route), and (3) elimination of "poorly performing" solutions. Survivor solutions are then permitted to mutate and cross-breed and compete further. Ultimately, the most desirable solution is selected from the set of all generated solutions. Note that there is no guarantee that all possible solutions are explored; and GAs, while quite efficient, cannot ensure that the winning solution is the single best choice.

Fuzzy Logic

Fuzzy logic is not a data analysis technique. It is a method of handling data permitting relative rather than crisp definitions, and as a result, it is particularly suited to medical applications. One of the interesting ironies of medical practice is that its practitioners strive for objectivity and precision while dealing with data that are inherently imprecise. Fuzzy logic has proven to be well suited to a variety of industrial applications and fuzzy control strategies are, in many cases, more efficient than traditional alternatives. For example, fuzzy control systems are used in elevator control, intelligent sensors, climate control, and image stabilization in video cameras, to name just a few (Fig. 19-5).

Fuzzy mathematics permits rigorous manipulation of terms like "too warm" or "very fast." It has many logical applications in medicine. Medical physiology is largely built around flexible, feedback control loops within the body, and yet our treatment strategies tend to be modeled on traditional "on/off" control circuits. For example, compare two strategies to control blood pressure with an intravenous infusion. The traditional approach involves a stepwise dose change based on blood pressure response, and is typically controlled by a bedside nurse. An automated fuzzy control strategy might use a rule like "increase the blood pressure medication rapidly if the blood pressure is very high," or "decrease the blood pressure infusion slowly if the blood pressure is decreasing slowly." Using this approach, the medication is titrated continuously rather than in a stepwise fashion (Fig. 19-6). Automated, feedback-controlled infusion devices of this kind have been shown to be effective and safe.

Fuzzy logic control systems are easy to design and modify. More importantly, unlike NNs, the

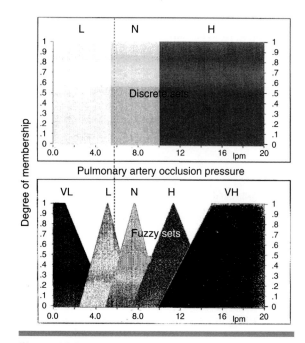

Figure 19-5
Medical clinicians are typically taught in terms of absolutes, such as the low, normal, and high pulmonary artery occlusion pressures in the top frame, whereas the overlapping "fuzzy" descriptions (very low, low, normal, and so on) in the bottom frame are better representations of reality.

logical constructs used in these systems are easy to describe, and closely approximate the thinking processes used in clinical decision making.

Machine Learning

Machine learning algorithms create classification schemes by searching through data for relevant patterns and generating rules that can be evaluated and understood by an observer. Machine learning algorithms require the creation of a data set with independent and dependent variables. The machine learning algorithm is then used to explore the data for relationships between the independent and dependent variables. For example, a machine learning approach might be used to evaluate the relative contribution of diet, age, smoking history, serum

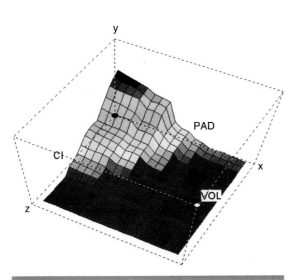

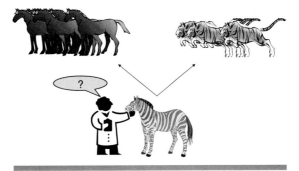

Figure 19-7
A case-based reasoning system has an accumulated database of previous cases and "solutions" that can be referred to for the solution of a new case, which is then, itself, added to the case base.

Figure 19-6
A theoretical "control surface" for an automatic fluid resuscitation machine where the volume infusion rate (y axis) increases as the patients cardiac index (CI) and pulmonary artery pressure (PAD) decrease.

cholesterol, and homocysteine level to the development of coronary artery disease.

Case-Based Reasoning

Case-based reasoning is a method of arriving at solutions by analogy and is very similar to the way in which experts reason when confronted with a new or challenging medical case (Fig. 19-7). A case consists of a series of attributes, and a series of representative cases are accumulated into a case base. The case base can then be examined by the use of probes or test cases (to find all cases in the database like the test case).

Case-based reasoning is well suited to the derivation of solutions when there are discontinuities in the case base. Case-based reasoning might be used to find cases similar to a hypothetical, newly presenting, and undiagnosed patient with rapidly evolving high fever, respiratory symptoms, and diarrhea, such as the symptoms of severe acute respiratory syndrome.

New diseases such as Hanta virus, AIDS, and Legionnaire's disease are discovered through a process analogous to case-based reasoning. While a case database might not contain a case with a specific constellation of conditions, case-based systems can extrapolate from other patients with similar histories. Case-based reasoning simulates the reasoning processes of an expert who has a large catalogue stored in his brain and can rapidly recall analogous cases.

Belief Networks

The power of Bayes Rule has been exploited to develop extremely powerful, readily understood learning algorithms known as Bayesian networks or belief networks (Fig. 19-8). They have been used for military applications such as the rapid identification of incoming military targets (missiles, aircraft, vessels) and deployment of counterattacks, and to assist computer software support staff. In the latter application, probability trees are constructed describing the potential sources of a customer problem. The initial design of a belief network requires the configuration of a tree of nodes describing the relationship of variables to an outcome. For example, one could construct a belief network describing the probabilities that a patient with ECG changes, chest pain and

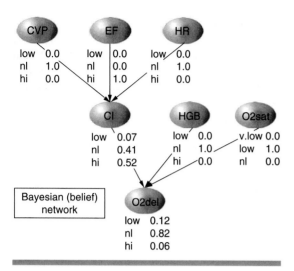

Figure 19-8
A belief network uses probabilities of related inputs to determine the likelihood of a given output.

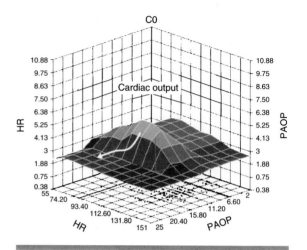

Figure 19-9
Data visualization can be used to show a large number of summarized data points (in this case sets of heart rate, pulmonary artery occlusion pressure and cardiac output) in a single view, thereby revealing important trends.

CHF has an acute myocardial infarction. The initial network could be "primed" with an expert's assignment of probabilities and then subsequently tuned with real values accumulated over time from a live database.

Data Visualization

Data visualization is a term used to describe the intelligent depiction of information using tools like proximity, grouping, shape, color, animation, and other techniques to enhance the comprehension of data by a viewer. There has not been a great deal of work done with medical data visualization, and most of what has been done is in fields like radiology. It is possible, however, to use visualization techniques to enhance the comprehension of relationships among data elements (Fig. 19-9).

Intelligent Algorithms in Medicine

There are a variety of data management tools that have become available over the past decade. They vary in their suitability to a given task, the degree to which the solution is understandable (transparent or opaque) and the ease of configurability. It is unlikely that intelligent software will replace the clinician in

the way that the original medical expert systems were conceived, rather these systems are more likely to act as intelligent assistants for specialized, complicated problems, and are generally intended to enhance the performance of a human expert. Safety has always been a concern and acted as a relative brake on the adoption of new technologies in medicine. Paradoxically, fuzzy control systems and NNs are being used in automated trains and elevators, helicopters, and even spacecraft, where the safety of more than one individual is often at risk.

It is reasonable to make some predictions about the ways in which these technologies will find their way into medical practice. NNs and fuzzy systems are particularly useful for waveform analysis. They will be integrated into bedside monitors and continuously analyze waveforms for known patterns (cardiac ischemia, hypovolemia). Fuzzy controllers will be integrated into bedside devices such as fluid and medication infusion devices, mechanical ventilators, and dialysis machines.

Belief networks and NNs will be used in the development of smart alarms that integrate multiple data streams (hemodynamics, laboratory data, other monitors), which display event probability (e.g., myocardial infarction). Case-based reasoning, machine learning algorithms, and visualization tools can be used to analyze information from large data stores. Data visualization tools will be designed to allow the clinician to interrogate and analyze significant trends in an individual patient or patient populations at a glance.

Data-driven decision support tools are required to permit the busy clinician (physician, nurse, respiratory therapist) to function more efficiently, caring for more patients more safely in much the same way that these same tools have been used to enhance the efficiency of business applications. Modern assembly lines have become more productive and make fewer errors than ever before, partly through the application of automated processes. Robotics has been another key driver in the improved efficiency of modern assembly lines.

Robotics in Medicine

Key Points

- Robotic devices are currently large, and largely untested in medical care.
- Surgical robots are beginning to come into use in several specific surgical procedures.
- Robotic devices have been designed to allow clinicians to "virtually" round on patients.
- Robotic technology can also be used in laboratory automation, drug delivery from pharmacy to bedside, and to augment the lifting power of healthcare personnel during patient care.

Robotic devices have the potential to radically change the delivery of healthcare, in much the same way that robotic assembly lines changed the way in which cars are manufactured. Robotic devices have been built for a number of surgical applications, such as robotic "scrub nurses," robot-assisted stereotactic procedures, and robotic surgical procedures controlled from a console. A robotic scrub nurse can select requested instruments and deliver them to the surgeon using voice

recognition and learning algorithms. The robot can keep track of the number of instruments and learn the preferences of a given surgeon. Surgical robots have been used for cardiac, thoracic, bariatric, and urologic procedures. The surgical arms can perform procedures through small incisions. Software built into these systems can eliminate tremor and, by synchronizing with the heart or diaphragm, reduce cardiac or respiratory artifact (Fig. 19-10).

Robotic "remote-presence" machines can be used to allow a physician to "visit" patients through telepresence. The physician can be off-site and still see and interact with a patient using the robot mounted camera and microphone. This approach could be used to permit a physician to round on

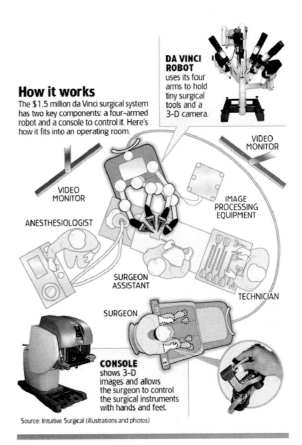

How it works
The $1.5 million da Vinci surgical system has two key components: a four-armed robot and a console to control it. Here's how it fits into an operating room.

DA VINCI ROBOT uses its four arms to hold tiny surgical tools and a 3-D camera.

VIDEO MONITOR

VIDEO MONITOR

ANESTHESIOLOGIST

IMAGE PROCESSING EQUIPMENT

SURGEON ASSISTANT

TECHNICIAN

SURGEON

CONSOLE shows 3-D images and allows the surgeon to control the surgical instruments with hands and feet.

Source: Intuitive Surgical (illustrations and photos)

Figure 19-10
Operating robots permit the surgeon to sit at a remote console and operate through small incisions.

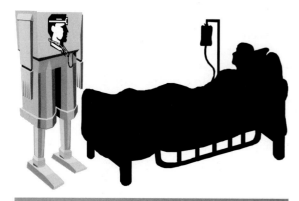

Figure 19-11
Robots are being used for "virtual rounding," allowing the clinician to be more efficient in care delivery.

patients at several sites from a central console in an office or home (Fig. 19-11).

Robots have been designed to deliver drugs from a central pharmacy to a nursing unit. Robotic lifts can lift and move patients, which might otherwise occupy the efforts of several nurses simultaneously. One can conceive of robotic transport devices to move patients around within a hospital facility from site to site, as for radiographic studies.

Alternatively, diagnostic, robotically delivered technologies can come to the bedside, as with a robotically performed echocardiographic study. In this case, an untrained individual can bring a robotic echocardiographic device to the patient and perform the echo examination, perhaps with remote direction by an echo technician or cardiologist.

Finally, robotic devices have also been de-signed to assist in physical therapy, permitting continuous feedback as to the level of physical effort used by the patient to manipulate a robotic arm.

■ Other Technologies

Key points

■ New technologies for tracking have made package delivery and trucking much more efficient, and these same technologies can be applied to the management of patient care.

■ Nanotechnology is an area with great promise for the future, but one in which there has been a great deal of hype it is unclear what the future will actually hold.

Many new electronic technologies are beginning to be deployed in hospitals after having proved themselves in other environments. Radio frequency ID tags (Chap. 4) and bar codes are well suited to inventory control as well as to the correct matching of patient and therapy. These technologies can be used to match drugs to patients as well as ensure that the correct blood products are given to the correct patient.

Tracking

Tracking software and hardware has substantially increased the efficiency of a variety of industries. Truckers are tracked using Global Positioning System. Fedex and united parcel service (UPS) packages are tracked from point of departure through point of delivery to the minute. The technologies that permit this are be-coming available in hospitals and will inevitably be applied to staff and patient tracking.

For example, it is extremely valuable to be able to track patients through the perioperative period and manage preop, prep, surgical, recovery, and intensive care areas based on actual utilization. This permits dynamic reassignment of cases and support services as indicated by actual demand rather than a quickly outdated paper schedule. Administrators, families, anesthesiologists, surgeons, and ancillary personnel can monitor information specific to their needs using automated tracking technology (Fig. 19-12).

There are other new productivity technologies that can be used to facilitate communications within a hospital, such as voice communicators using wireless network connections (voice over Internet protocol).

Nanotechnology

Nanotechnology is undoubtedly the next big thing. It will have wide ranging implications for medicine, including the development and delivery of drugs, the detection of disease states, and the treatment of same.

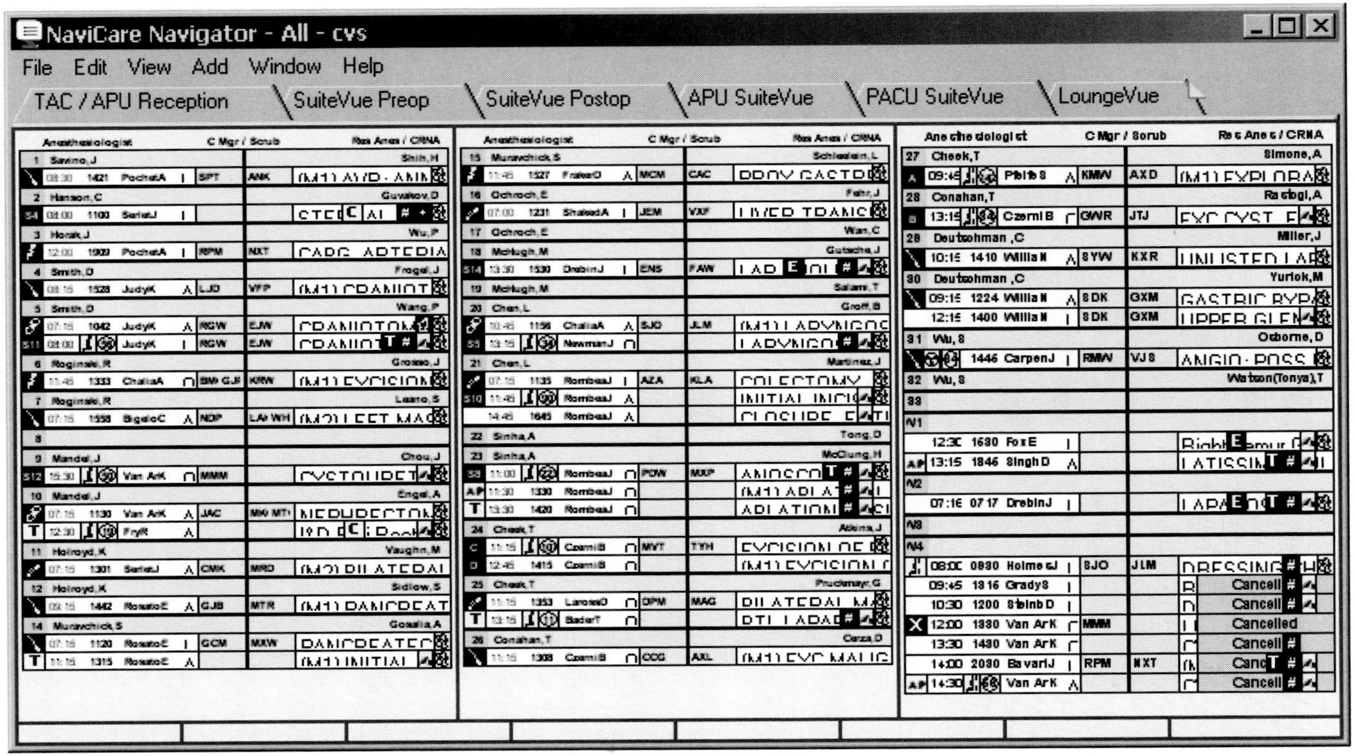

Figure 19-12

Tracking software is used to follow patients and resources as they move through critical areas such as the OR and ICU tracking software is used to follow patients and resources as they move through critical areas such as the OR and ICU (with permission of Hill-Rom, Navicare.)

What we conceive of as a drug is essentially a single molecule with a sophisticated but limited repertoire. Tomorrow's smart, nanotechnology-based drugs might be programmable machines with a range of "sensory," "decision-making," and "effector" capabilities. They may only become active only when they reach their intended targets, thereby attaining almost complete specificity of action. Groups of these drugs could work interactively using built-in programs to achieve the desired effect.

It will probably be possible to create nanoscale surgical instruments and cameras as well. Japanese engineers have made a nanoscale bull (Fig. 19-13) as well as a nanoscale spring. Similarly, Cornell scientists have created a rotor one-fifth the size of a red blood cell.

Conclusion

Many of the new technologies described in this chapter have been adapted for use in other industries with significant benefits in the quality and efficiency with which products are manufactured. Medicine has traditionally thought of itself as a high-quality, human-centered industry and very resistant to automation. The productivity and financial pressures operating in our world have become great enough that automation is inevitable. The difficulty will be distinguishing between automation for automation's sake and applications that improve the process and safety of care.

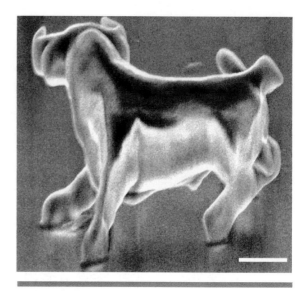

Figure 19-13
Nanoscale technology is coming of age as demonstrated by this nanoscale polymer bull which is the size of a red blood cell.

Suggested Readings

Desouza KC. *Managing Knowledge with Artificial Intelligence: An Introduction with Guidelines for Nonspecialists.* Westport: Quorum Books, 2002.
Schraft RD, Schmierer G. *Service Robots.* Natick, MA AK Peters, 2000.
Tufte ER. *Envisioning Information.* Graphics Press, 1990.
Tufte ER. *Visual Explanations: Images and Quantities, Evidence and Narrative.* Graphics Press, 1997.
Tufte ER. *The Visual Display of Quantitative Information,* 2nd ed. Graphics Press, Cheshire, Connecticut, 2001.

20 | Conclusion

▪ Conclusion

As we move into the twenty-first century, the promises of medicine are enormous, but so are the challenges and disparities. New technologies and therapies are developed every day, but so do the cost pressures. It is clear that medicine will need to undergo the same degree of retooling that other industries, such as the automotive and financial industries have, in order to remain viable.

Computers and computerized devices will clearly be integral to medicine's survival in its current form. Both President George Bush and Senator Hillary Clinton have referred to the computerized provider order entry (CPOE) as essential to improved medical care at lower cost, so the message has clearly gotten to the highest levels of government. The adoption of tools such as CPOEs and electronic health records has proceeded slowly, however, despite a clear-cut consensus on the part of insurers, providers, and patients.

There are a variety of barriers that need to be negotiated before these tools become the norm. Privacy concerns are significant and grow with each new revelation of data loss by large companies and financial institutions. The implementation of the Healthcare Insurance Portability and Accountability Act (HIPAA) legislation has hit the industry like the Y2K "sea change," however, and privacy protection is improving.

The medical software industry is nowhere near mature, and clinicians have been appropriately conservative in their adoption of products like CPOEs that have failed dramatically in some cases, such as Cedars-Sinai. There are, however, notable success stories and commercial vendors are delivering better products with improved sensitivity to the workflow issues inherent in converting to computerized ordering and record keeping.

The money needed to computerize is also needed at many institutions for infrastructure maintenance or to bring the physical plant into compliance with regulatory requirements. It is increasingly clear, however, that providers that are unable to become more efficient will fall increasingly behind more successful competitors. Computer supported medical care is like a claw or an eyeball: an evolutionary development that confers a competitive edge in an ecosystem under pressure.

Computer science and medical science have traditionally had little to say to one another. While there are a few outstanding medical informatics programs, such as those at Stanford, Vanderbilt, and Columbia, medical clinicians, be they physicians, nurses, or ancillary personnel, have had very little education about computers during their training. Happily, this is changing rapidly, with the integration of computers and digital devices into medical school curricula.

Recent trainees are much more comfortable with computers, software, and digital data. As a result, they are much more likely to accept well-designed products and integrate them into care delivery. While it is not yet clear exactly how medicine will change with computerization, the advent of technologies such as telemedicine, faster networking, and virtual reality give tantalizing glimpses of what it might look like. One needs only to look at how rapidly the world has changed with the advent of the Internet to understand how quickly the process will happen with sufficient momentum, and many things suggest that that time has come.

INDEX